Triathlon
Workout Planner

Triathlon Workout Planner

John Mora

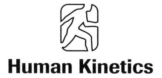

Human Kinetics

Library of Congress Cataloging-in-Publication Data

Mora, John, 1964-
  Triathlon workout planner / John M. Mora
      p. cm.
  Includes bibliographical references and index.
  ISBN 0-7360-5905-9 (soft cover)
  1. Triathlon--Training. I. Title.
  GV1060.73.M674 2004
  796.42'57--dc22

                              2005027060

ISBN-10: 0-7360-5905-9

ISBN-13: 978-0-7360-5905-3

Copyright © 2006 by John M. Mora

The Web addresses cited in this text were current as of August 8, 2005, unless otherwise noted.

Acquisitions Editor: Martin Barnard; **Developmental Editor:** Amanda M. Eastin; **Assistant Editors:** Mandy Maiden and Christine Horger; **Copyeditor:** Kathy Calder; **Proofreader:** John Wentworth; **Indexer:** Nancy Ball; **Permission Manager:** Carly Breeding; **Graphic Designer:** Fred Starbird; **Graphic Artist:** Tara Welsch; **Photo Manager:** Dan Wendt; **Cover Designer:** Keith Blomberg; **Photographer (cover):** © Human Kinetics; **Printer:** Sheridan Books

Human Kinetics books are available at special discounts for bulk purchase. Special editions or book excerpts can also be created to specification. For details, contact the Special Sales Manager at Human Kinetics.

Printed in the United States of America   10   9   8   7   6   5

The paper in this book is certified under a sustainable forestry program.

Human Kinetics
Web site: www.HumanKinetics.com

United States: Human Kinetics
P.O. Box 5076
Champaign, IL 61825-5076
800-747-4457
e-mail: humank@hkusa.com

Canada: Human Kinetics
475 Devonshire Road, Unit 100
Windsor, ON N8Y 2L5
800-465-7301 (in Canada only)
e-mail: info@hkcanada.com

Europe: Human Kinetics
107 Bradford Road
Stanningley
Leeds LS28 6AT, United Kingdom
+44 (0)113 255 5665
e-mail: hk@hkeurope.com

Australia: Human Kinetics
57A Price Avenue
Lower Mitcham, South Australia 5062
08 8372 0999
e-mail: info@hkaustralia.com

New Zealand: Human Kinetics
P.O. Box 80
Torrens Park, South Australia 5062
0800 222 062
e-mail: info@hknewzealand.com

Planning your triathlon training takes discipline, energy, and, most of all, passion.

Two people planning their lives together takes all that and more.

To Linda, who gives me more than I could ask for every day.

Contents

Preface

Have you ever had the experience of striving for something and finding out down the road that you don't have the time, energy, or motivation to follow through? Or worse, have you killed yourself physically, mentally, and spiritually to accomplish a goal, only to realize that you didn't enjoy one single bit of it?

If you really want to get fit and accomplish your triathlon goals, you've got to be realistic and organized, and you've got to focus on the workouts that are going to help you cross the finish line with a strong sprint.

Realistic means something different to everyone. What may be realistic for one person is totally insane for another. All of us have unique responsibilities in terms of work, family, and social commitments. The trick is to determine a commitment level (and race distance and goal) that will contribute to—not detract from—a balanced lifestyle. Then you've got to put all the pieces together to make that happen. *Triathlon Workout Planner* is designed to help you do just that so that you can train intelligently and effectively within your personal time constraints.

Part I of this book provides you with some valuable information to help you get started. You'll find out how to determine the best race goal for you, manage your time and set priorities, find workout structures that will fit with your busy schedule, and create a master training plan that is uniquely suited to your training needs and goals. In addition, you'll be introduced to some key concepts that will significantly improve your chances of success, both in terms of making the most of what time you have and achieving your race goal.

Part II introduces you to some important tools that will help you train more intelligently and more effectively, resulting in improved performances. You'll find out how to use heart rate training for your current fitness level and adjust your target zones for sport-specific triathlon training. Concepts like key workouts and abiding by the 80/20 rule will help you stay on track and make leaps-and-bounds progress toward your goal. I've provided descriptions of intervals, bricks, and a host of other key workouts to help you pick and choose what works best for you. These race-proven training structures will directly contribute to your success on race day.

The sample workouts in part III will give you a good indication of how you can structure your individual training plan. Customized for each of the four most popular triathlon distances, these sample workouts provide a snapshot of what typical training might encompass, as well as a tapering schedule that will help you recover and be fresh for that big day.

PART I

Plan for Success

Setting your priorities, managing your time well, and creating a plan are the first steps necessary in achieving your triathlon goal. By learning how to plan and train well within your time constraints, you'll maximize the efficiency of your workouts while maintaining balance in your life. Most of all, these tools will bring greater clarity and focus to your training, giving you the best shot at achieving your triathlon goal, whatever it may be. So roll up your wet-suit sleeves, and let's get to work.

CHAPTER 1

Priority Checklist

Admit it. You've caught the triathlon bug. You're officially a tri-geek. If you're reading this book, chances are that you're pretty serious about training. But training for the sake of training can eventually lead to burnout, and triathletes have gone down that path far too often through the years.

What you need is a plan—a good plan that incorporates your personal goals within a realistic framework, while making the most efficient use of your time. As you set forth on your quest for personal triathlon glory, the first order of business is to determine where your heart is. Selecting your goals shouldn't be like shooting at random targets. It's a process of examining yourself to determine objectives that get your heart racing in more than the cardiovascular way.

The key to accomplishing what you want to accomplish in your triathlon training is simple. Like most things in life, it's a matter of setting your priorities and creating a smart and realistic plan around them. In this chapter, we'll begin our journey toward more efficient and effective triathlon training by determining your goals, assessing your current fitness on several levels, and looking at which race distances will suit you best. We'll also explore the benefits of two training tools: a seasonal racing calendar and a training log.

SETTING GOALS

I recently had an unpleasant experience while taking my weekly long run. After struggling both mentally and physically for the first 6 miles of my 12-mile run, I came to a disheartening conclusion: I didn't want to run. I kept going, mainly because I was 6 miles away from my house (which is the greatest benefit of out-and-back courses—you can't get home unless you finish the run). There was no physical reason why the run had been so hard for me. In the next few days I recovered well, faster than usual, in fact. But after looking over all the factors, checking my training log, and

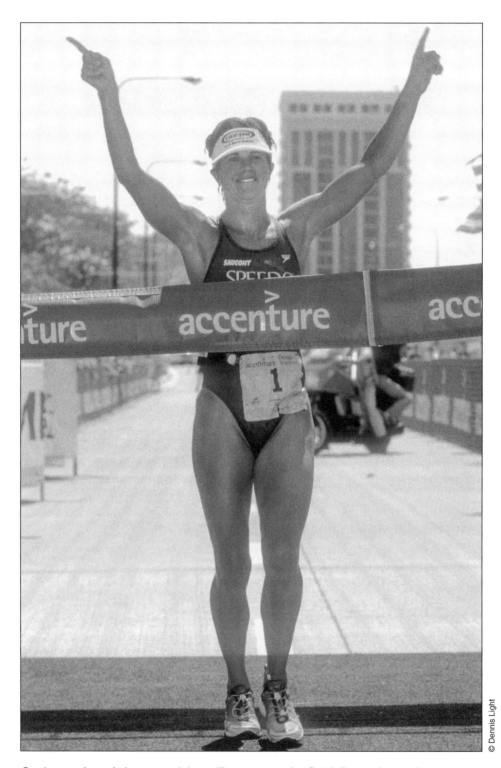

© Dennis Light

Setting goals early in your training will get you to the finish line with a smile on your face.

examining any variables that had changed in my training program recently, I realized what the problem was: I had no goal.

Perhaps you are the type of triathlete who trains for the sake of training. If so, you are a true triathlete, having gone through the three steps of tri-evolution—from newbie to weekend warrior to tri-geek. I personally find it difficult to train for any period longer than 30 minutes or to elevate my heart rate above 150 for any length of time unless there's a clear, tangible purpose to my training. Having recently decided to skip a late summer half-Ironman race because of a conflict in work schedule, I was faced with a 12-mile run that had no purpose. The result was loss of energy and motivation, which manifested itself in physical discomfort and fatigue.

The true tri-geek swims, bikes, and runs for the sake of training and for the benefits, both physical and mental, of exerting the body in such a beautifully exhaustive way. The tri-geek trains for the sheer pleasure of it. However, every triathlete, no matter how dedicated or self-motivated, will benefit from setting a goal and designing a training program based on that target. Simply put, your long-term goal should be your ultimate destination, driven by your heart's desire and supported by short-term goals.

Short-Term Goals

As you begin to think about your goal or about a series of objectives (such as completing multiple races in a certain cumulative time), it's easy to fall into the trap of failing to set the short-term goals that will get you there. Although your ultimate long-term goal is the destination at the top of the ladder, you've got to climb the rungs; that is, accomplish the interim steps you need to reach higher and higher levels of performance.

You can also think of short-term goals as the links in a chain that will lead you to where you want to go. Short-term goals focus your attention for only several days, weeks, or months. Often there are several short-term goals for each long-term goal. By setting realistic, measurable, and motivational short-term goals that link together throughout a plan, you'll be well on your way to crossing that finish line with a huge smile on your face.

Without really thinking about it, all of us set short-term goals for the normal, mundane tasks we have to do every day. We go to the store, drive to work, and take the kids to school. Every time we make a decision to do something, the subconscious mind takes over, and we get it done, sometimes without even remembering we did it. Although swimming, biking, and running may not fall under the same category as your daily errands, setting short-term goals will help provide focus and clarity to your daily and weekly triathlon training.

The qualities and characteristics of your short-term goals for triathlon training are perhaps even more important than those of your long-term goals. The time you spend establishing these small, intermediate steps is more critical to your success than anything else you will do in the early stages of your training. That's because the early stages of training make you susceptible to injury and burnout if your goals are initially set too high. But when you take the time to establish short-term goals tempered by a solid grasp of your current fitness and by proven training principles, you can hit your long-term target with a bull's-eye.

You must first understand what makes for good short-term goals. As you begin mulling over some of the intermediate steps you need to take in working toward your target, make sure your short-term triathlon goals have these characteristics:

• **Specific.** Make sure you set specific benchmarks you can measure. Otherwise, how will you know when you've achieved your goal? Benchmarks need not be complicated, just specific enough that you can tangibly know when you have met the goal and then reward yourself for the accomplishment. For example, working out at least five days a week for one hour a day would be a valid short-term goal, because it provides clear benchmarks that specify the frequency and duration of the workout. Conversely, "working out consistently" is nonspecific—it doesn't provide the detail and measurement of achievement you need to motivate yourself to train properly.

• **Realistic.** You should establish inner-based performance goals—those based on the things you can control—as opposed to setting outcome-based goals, which depend on many uncontrollable variables. The goal of working out five days a week for an hour a day is realistic, because you can control how many times a week you train and for how many hours. However, setting a goal of coming in first during a competitive bike club group ride may only lead to discouragement if you don't yet have the fitness level and cycling skills to pull it off. You may find that success at achieving a series of inner-based performance goals will often lead to outward achievements, such as placing in your age-group.

• **Prioritized.** Your short-term goals should focus first and foremost on your training weaknesses; that is, the areas that are most troublesome for you. For example, if swimming is your weakness, setting a short-term goal of swimming at least three to five times a week is warranted. If overall consistency is a problem, setting a specific number of hours per week or workouts per week is best. Many triathletes make the mistake of catering to their strengths and ignoring their weaknesses in training. Prioritize your goals so that they address your greatest needs and shore up your most bothersome weaknesses.

Document your goals to help bring focus to your plan. Use the planning tools provided in this book to write down your short-term goals, but also use daily reminders such as scheduling time in your daily or weekly planner or computer contact manager. You simply can't overdo this aspect of goal-setting. In fact, writing down your triathlon short-term goals on a small piece of paper or index card that you carry with you during the day is a good visual cue and a subtle reminder at various times of the day, when you're not working out.

Long-Term Goals

Your long-term goal is possibly what you had foremost in your mind when you bought this book. Perhaps it's completing your first triathlon or maybe your first Ironman-distance race. Maybe it's completing a series of multisport events. Set a long-term goal that is challenging but realistic. Most important of all, take some time to ensure your goal is compatible with your priorities and your work and family obligations.

Let's face it—fitting triathlon training into a busy lifestyle can be a huge challenge. Unless you're independently wealthy, have few family obligations, and have plenty of time for swimming, cycling, and running, triathlon training requires some good balancing skills. In the coming chapters you'll find information about efficient time management and the tools you need to make this balancing act work for you, provided that you've established a realistic long-term goal to set you on the right course from the outset.

Long-term goals share the attributes mentioned under short-term goals, with some important added factors:

• **Visionary.** I've stressed the importance of being grounded in reality when setting goals, but it's just as important to think outside the box when it comes to setting a triathlon target. If you're a triathlon veteran who has raced sprint or Olympic distances for a while, have you considered making the jump to a half-Ironman or Ironman distance? What about completing a series of races in a cumulative time? How about a particularly challenging race on a tough course? When you ponder your goal, allow yourself the freedom to consider the many possibilities.

• **Believable.** You should temper your vision with a belief that your long-term goal is plausible. It's what *you* believe you can accomplish—not what others may think. You know best what you can personally commit to and achieve, so make sure that belief is there from the onset.

• **Inspiring.** Plenty of months of training ahead will not be easy. Although triathlon training and racing count among the most fun times in my life, I can recall just as many long, hot, bumpy bike rides and equally nightmarish runs. What kept me going was a race goal that I just couldn't give up on. Make sure your long-term goal will inspire and motivate you for the months of tough training to come.

Table 1.1 shows some examples of how to use a planning tool to create a road map to your triathlon goals. Use the blank goal planner from table 12.1 (see p. 130) to help you set your short- and long-term goals.

Table 1.1   Goal Planner Examples

Long-term goal	Deadline or metric
Finish first half-Ironman triathlon.	(Race date)
Short-term goals	**Deadline or metric**
Work out at least five days each week.	Start now.
Do Wednesday night group rides.	Start this Wednesday.
Run 25 miles (40 kilometers) per week with one long run on Sundays.	Start this week.
Participate in at least four organized century rides this summer.	(Four ride dates listed)
Run half-marathon later this summer as a training race.	(Race date)
Get up one hour earlier to do Masters group swim workouts at the YMCA on Monday, Wednesday, and Friday of each week.	Start this Monday.
Save $50 per paycheck for a new triathlon bike.	$1,000 by (date).
Join local triathlon club.	Go to new member meeting on (date).

ASSESSING FITNESS LEVEL

In order to get where you want to go, it's vital to know where you are. When you plan for your triathlon goal, one of the first critical steps will be to ask some questions about your present overall fitness. Now that you've documented your long-term goals and the steps you need to take to reach them, it's time to take a good hard look at the current status of your greatest resource—your body.

The three primary components of fitness are cardiovascular conditioning, strength, and flexibility. Although most triathletes focus on cardio, these three components in their entirety define total fitness. When assessing your fitness level, strength and flexibility must be taken into consideration. Concentrating on cardiovascular conditioning in endurance sports without giving some thought to strength training will leave you with an area of imbalance in your exercise regimen, which could cause you injury. By the same token, if you concentrate on strength training without any heed to cardiovascular conditioning, you'll lack the endurance for almost any sustained activity.

Let's take a look at each of the three components separately and determine some key assessment tests and questions that may give you some insight into your current fitness level. Armed with this information, you can make adjustments to your goals and be better prepared to plan your training.

Cardiovascular Fitness

Cardiovascular fitness is the ability of the lungs to provide oxygen to the blood and the ability of the heart to transport the oxygenated blood to the cells of the body. Basically, it's your ability to sustain an activity for an extended period of time. There are several methods to assess your cardiovascular fitness, but I've chosen two that stand out as particularly good measures associated with endurance sports. Some measures are more precise than others, but you must determine a fairly accurate assessment of your fitness level so that your training begins at a pace, intensity, and duration that is right for you.

$\dot{V}O_2max$

The term $\dot{V}O_2max$ is a cardiorespiratory measurement that quantifies your body's ability to deliver oxygen to cells in one minute—the higher the $\dot{V}O_2max$, the fitter the athlete. Simply put, $\dot{V}O_2max$ represents the maximum amount of oxygen that can be removed from circulating blood and used by the working tissues during a specified period. For example, elite cyclists and other endurance athletes may have very high $\dot{V}O_2max$ rates of 70 to 80 ml/kg/min. A fit triathlete who trains and races on a regular basis probably has a value in the 35 to 50 range. Sedentary people usually have values of less than 20.

How do you determine your $\dot{V}O_2max$? If you had the time and money to perform a sophisticated $\dot{V}O_2max$ treadmill test in a human performance sports laboratory equipped with computerized gadgets attached to your body, you could get a precise measurement of your body's ability to deliver oxygen during the stress of a triathlon. However, since this type of testing isn't available to most people, you can roughly estimate your $\dot{V}O_2max$ based on the Cooper test for $\dot{V}O_2max$.

To estimate your $\dot{V}O_2max$ using the Cooper test, you must complete a 12-minute run on a course measured in meters. Ideally you'll want to run on a 400-meter track, with signs for every 100 meters. Run as many meters as you can for 12 minutes, rounding off to the nearest 100 meters. Use the following formula to calculate your $\dot{V}O_2max$:

(Distance covered in meters − 504.9) ÷ 44.73 = your $\dot{V}O_2max$.

To help you assess your current fitness level based on your $\dot{V}O_2max$, table 1.2 provides average normative values for different age groups, categorizing them from "very poor" to "superior." Comparing your $\dot{V}O_2max$

If you have not been strength training consistently, chances are you have some chinks in your triathlon armor. You can pinpoint areas that are weak in a number of ways, including standardized strength tests in which you work major muscle groups to exhaustion or perform abdominal exercises, push-ups, or any number of strength exercises for a set time (or even for one repetition). You can measure your results against a table to find out your overall strength score in that muscle group. Doing these tests with a strength-training expert can tell you which muscles or muscle groups you should work on.

A personal trainer can put you through a testing regimen and determine key areas of weakness that you may need to shore up to improve your swimming, cycling, and running muscles and your overall strength. A common sense alternative would be to focus on specific areas where you have had difficulty in the past, evidenced by injury or poor performance. For example, if you have difficulty in generating power during hilly triathlon bike courses, you can include some leg presses, lunges, gluteus kickbacks, and squats in your workout. If you've had knee injuries, strengthening the ligaments and muscles around your knees with leg extensions (provided you are now healthy) should be part of your program.

The triathlon imposes many forces on many parts of your body, making it the ultimate cross-training sport. As you assess your strength, make sure you create a program for yourself that takes into account this variety of forces by including all the major and minor muscle groups, as well as the all-important core. Plan your strength training to coordinate with your higher-intensity endurance work so that no part of your body is unduly taxed. Don't do leg presses or squats the day before or after a hard track workout. Alternate muscle groups so that you give them plenty of rest between workouts (for example, work the lower body one session, the upper body the next).

Flexibility Fitness

As a whole, we triathletes tend to be a tight group. If we aren't grabbing our Achilles tendon in pain, we're probably massaging our aching hamstrings from yesterday's track workout. We also tend to be somewhat imbalanced muscularly—big quads, weak hamstrings, and the back imbalances that can develop from all the hours hunching over the aero bars. Stretching not only helps keep muscles loose but also improves body alignment and balance. Ironically, we tend to be quite lazy when it comes to stretching. For example, I rarely stretch before a run, and only occasionally will I do a few wall push-ups or toe touches after a run that's made my muscles ache.

Lately, however, I've been noticing the importance of stretching as my mileage goes up and the countdown before the upcoming fall Ironman season goes down. If you're like me, you'd rather just jump into your running shoes and head out on the trails before the sun goes down. But as I've grown older and less flexible, I've learned just how important my flexibility can be in preventing injury and improving my overall health.

Flexibility is the capacity of a joint to move through its full range of motion. If you are having difficulty achieving a full range of motion in a joint or sense tightness in a particular part of the body, chances are that you have flexibility issues—you may be knocking on the door of a sports injury.

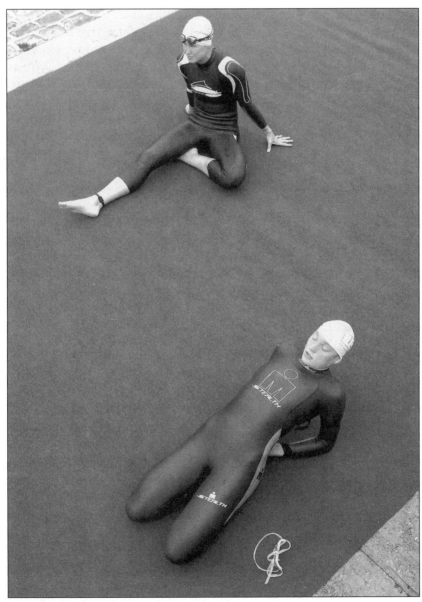

Stretching before a race can warm your body up and calm your mind down.

© Nigel Farrow

Even if you pinpoint no specific flexibility issues, including stretching or massage in your triathlon training plan will ensure better health and fitness (see chapter 2 for more information about stretching and the value of massage therapy). If you've read running books and subscribe to *Runner's World* or any other running publication, you've probably come across a lot of material on stretching. There are about as many stretching techniques and exercises for endurance athletes as there are sports drinks. However, most fitness experts recommend two methods of stretching: static and dynamic.

In the past, the type of stretching technique most sports therapists recommended was static stretching. This is a conservative technique—traditionally accepted as safe and effective—that involves a slow, gradual elongation through a full range of motion. In more basic terms, you stretch a given area to a point of slight discomfort and hold it for a set period of time, usually 15 to 30 seconds. An example is doing the wall push-up after a run, which holds a stretch in the hamstrings and calves.

Stretching promotes blood flow, helps flush lactic acid from your muscles, and promotes balance and good posture. Static stretching can be particularly beneficial when you have sore muscles after exercise, providing some relief to tight and taxed muscles. The slow, patient method of static stretching also promotes relaxation and stress relief.

However, nowadays many triathletes and weekend warriors are embracing more dynamic stretching methods, such as yoga and Pilates, that promote flexibility through active movement (but not beyond your normal range of motion). Dynamic stretches can also be done in sets or reps, as you would do in a strength-training session. These more dynamic methods have the added benefit of improving strength and core fitness, as well as having a warming effect on muscles and joints.

The optimum stretching technique has always been—and probably always will be—a matter of controversy. Since the added benefit of dynamic stretching is warming up muscles, I've found it helpful to do dynamic stretching *before* training, and then relax into static stretching as a recovery session *after* a hard workout.

CHOOSING A RACE DISTANCE

The triathlon distance you choose for your goal will have a huge impact on your schedule and family commitments during the next few months to a year. You may already have a distance in mind, but before you set it in stone, consider these factors.

• **Time commitment.** Unless you're financially independent and have no family, chances are you have some commitments that will be competing for your triathlon training time. Be realistic about how much time you'll be able to devote to triathlon training.

• **Physical limitations.** Is there anything that could possibly hold you back from committing to a specific distance? Do you have any past injuries that may prove to be a major obstacle when running long distances for the half-Ironman or Ironman events? Maybe you're not blessed with the perfect runner's body, or maybe you have difficulty swimming in open water for extended periods. There's no shame in testing the waters with a shorter distance and working up, if you think you are limited in any way.

• **Foundation.** If you're considering training for a half-Ironman or Ironman event, you should have a solid base of shorter triathlons or long-distance events in one or more of the three disciplines under your belt. Although many beginners have gone from sprint to Ironman within a year, it's best to progress from the shorter distances to the ultra events. Doing so establishes a fitness foundation over time that will make your path to success in the long events all the more safe and gratifying.

• **Desire.** What does your gut tell you is the best distance target to set for yourself? Above all else, you should enjoy your triathlon experience. Don't give in to peer pressure or outside expectations when choosing your target. Let your heart be your guide, and choose the distance that *you* want to try for.

Other factors unique to you may also play a part in your decision about a race distance. All these factors need to be given the appropriate weight and priority that only you can discern. Once you find the right distance that challenges you while keeping your life balanced, you'll find plenty of workout plans in part III to help take you to the finish line.

CREATING A SEASONAL CALENDAR

Creating a program with three or four goal-specific stages, each stage lasting from one to three months, is an important component of triathlon training. In addition to setting objectives that build on each other, changing your workout focus a few times a year makes sense, because you want to accomplish certain levels of fitness and skill and build on them sequentially. This variety also helps keep the mind fresh and the body challenged.

You can organize your training calendar in many different ways to achieve your goal. Generally, however, you should design it so that you do the following:

1. Start from a foundation of fitness and solidify it.
2. Begin developing speed, addressing specific weaknesses, and acquiring needed skills.
3. Focus on performance and prepare for the conditions and intensity of your event.
4. Give yourself needed rest (tapering) just before you hit the starting line.

Individualizing your race calendar is part of the fun of triathlon planning, so feel free to be creative and include the type of training that you feel will benefit you. For example, maybe triathlon is more of a social experience for you. In that case, you may want to plan a group run and ride season in which you focus on participating in a series of century rides and running races that you enjoy (and that will help you achieve your triathlon goal). Upcoming chapters will give you the knowledge and tools you need to create a seasonal training calendar that helps you meet your goals.

To introduce the structure for the workout plans provided in the book, here's a brief description of the training stages I'll refer to from time to time.

- **Base training.** Look at base training as the foundation on which everything else you do stands. This is a phase of training that—if executed properly—may take several months or an entire season. But the long-term rewards are injury prevention and greater performance. It's also worth noting that if your goal is merely to finish a race, your workouts may consist almost entirely of base training. That's fine. As long as you have a solid foundation, just finishing a race is a realistic goal. Base training consists mainly of long workouts done at a slow pace. Your focus should be on gradual total-mileage increases of no more than 10 percent per week, a rule that is especially crucial for running and helps avoid common overtraining injuries.

- **Speed, technique, and skills training (STS).** This is a training segment that allows you to begin building some competence in the areas of speed and technique. Speed improvement typically includes interval work or training specifically designed to increase your $\dot{V}O_2$max. Technique and skills training may include swim drills and transition work. This stage is also a prime time to work on any possible weaknesses. You will still be building your base and overall endurance while integrating workouts that introduce a higher level of stress to your body, in preparation for peak training.

- **Peak training.** Once you've established a solid base, done speed work, and tweaked your technique and skills, peak training can take you to the next level of performance. It is typically a short phase of high-intensity work that is totally aimed at your performing well for your race or goal. Bricks (sessions consisting of two or more disciplines) will be critical, as will other key workouts that focus on race performance.

- **Tapering.** This may be your most welcome stage of training after all that hard work. Tapering is a reduction of both intensity and workout duration that occurs a week or two before the event, depending on the race distance. Decreases in both mileage and distance during this stage will ensure that you are fresh, both mentally and physically, for your upcoming race goal. See chapter 3 for more discussion on tapering.

KEEPING A TRAINING LOG

If a written log hasn't been one of your training priorities, you're missing a valuable tool that will provide you with the kind of feedback you'll eventually need. Logs can help you in the following ways:

• **Injury prevention.** Sometimes we underestimate the training we've done. By analyzing actual workout totals and intensity, you can properly plan for needed rest and avoid overtraining that could lead to injury.

• **Personal triggers.** Did you ever have a really great workout and wonder why? Of course, everyone's had the opposite experience as well. Logs can help you decipher the enigma of your body and give clues to performance or weakness. They can help you see the best time of day to exercise, what to eat, what heart rate to target, how many hours of sleep you need—the possibilities are endless.

• **Workout planning.** Perhaps the greatest use of a log is as a planning tool for future training. By documenting many important variables, such as workout intensity, course, conditions, and how you felt, you'll be able to see what progress you have made and to plan the coming weeks and months appropriately. The log pages at the end of this book are designed to help you do that and more. You'll find many features on each page that relate specifically to some of the training methods and strategies outlined in the book, as well as plenty of opportunity for you to customize your logs. With a gold mine of data at your fingertips, collected from every workout recorded in your log, you'll be able to train efficiently toward your goal.

CHAPTER 2

Tri-Time Management

L ike any serious commitment, triathlon training requires a fairly sizable chunk of your time. As the popularity of multisports continues to grow, the demand for time-management strategies and practical ways to fit training into a busy lifestyle grows as well. In fact, the perception that it takes too much time to train properly for finishing a triathlon is one of the reasons many active people in the mainstream have not embraced the sport. Obviously, training for an Ironman-distance event requires a significant commitment of time and energy. However, the majority of triathlons in the sprint category require little more time than training for the typical Sunday morning 10K—if an exercise regimen is executed smartly and efficiently.

Whether you have a family, a demanding job, or other time limitations, managing your time well can mean the difference between crawling and sprinting to the finish line. In this chapter you'll learn not only how to make the most of your limited time but also how to be more flexible, efficient, and balanced regarding your energy level and triathlon lifestyle. Although making the best use of your training time is important, so is the rest of your life.

MAKING TIME

The first step in managing your training time is determining exactly where in your schedule triathlon training will fit. Creating blocks of time apportioned for your training not only creates a space in your schedule for training, but it also solidifies your commitment in your mind.

How much time will you have to block off on a weekly basis? Time spent training can vary according to your goal, training phase, and many other factors. Generally speaking, the longer the distance you are training for, the greater the range of time you must allow. Of course, the actual time you spend training for your race (or on training-related activities such as driving to the pool) will depend on unique factors such as proximity to a swimming pool, type of bike course, and running pace. I can make some generalizations about typical training weeks for various distances, based on my own experience and that of triathletes I've interviewed. Training for the sprint distance requires an estimated commitment of 8 to 12 hours per week, the Olympic distance 10 to 16 hours, the half-Ironman 14 to 25 hours, and the Ironman 20 to 35 hours.

If you have a set schedule that you can easily manipulate, apportioning training time may be a hassle-free process for you. A schedule that is inflexible and full of demands that are hard to anticipate may be your greatest challenge in time management. No matter what your life is like, here are a few keys to ensuring you make time for proper training.

• **Prioritize.** You've got 168 hours in a week. But when you subtract 7 hours of sleeping time per night, you've probably got somewhere in the neighborhood of 119 hours. That's it. Don't fool yourself into thinking that somehow, magically, you'll have more time than you have now without sacrificing something. Given your priorities and other commitments, you will most likely have to sacrifice some personal leisure, such as television time or curling up with that favorite book.

• **Get enough sleep.** During deep sleep your body repairs itself from all the hard training by secreting growth hormone. Growth hormone is one of the anabolic hormones needed for self-healing of muscle tissue. Over 50 percent of the body is muscle tissue, and hard training creates microtears that need repairing. Without proper sleep, the body does not secrete enough growth hormone to help muscles heal normally. Continued training without enough sleep will only add to your inability to recover. Bottom line, you need deep sleep, or else you will be working counterproductively.

• **Allow for commuting, preparation, and postworkout tasks.** When building training blocks into your weekly schedule, take into account all the necessary time you will spend on tasks in addition to the actual workout. For example, you have to allow for commuting time to and from the pool, bike prep time before your ride, and ample time to complete a run course without going beyond your intended intensity and pace. If your training will occur before work or during a lunch hour, you'll have to be extra careful about giving yourself ample wiggle room.

• **Be realistic.** The worst thing you can do is to create a weekly training schedule that imposes undue stress on you and your loved ones or puts your job or career in jeopardy. Take a few deep breaths, take a step back, and ask yourself, "Is this realistic?" If you find other important areas of your life deteriorating—romance, time with your kids, career opportunities—it probably means you're being unrealistic in the time you've apportioned to training.

FLEXIBLE SCHEDULING

Although I'm a big fan of planning and executing, there's truly something to be said for playing it by ear, particularly when it comes to such an unpredictable vessel as the human body. You may feel particularly good on a given bike ride and decide to push the pace or go longer. As long as you adjust any other training to accommodate for more recovery, there is absolutely nothing wrong with an impromptu change. Also, if you have a schedule that is not fixed, scheduling your training time on a flexible basis may work best for you, as long as you have the self-discipline to be vigilant about making sure those workouts regularly happen.

The mantra of flexibility is this: Listen to your body. When your body says, "I'm recovered and ready to run," then off you go. But when your legs cry, "Dude, no way," the flexible mind doesn't force its body out the door. Better to take the day off or seek an alternative cross-training activity to get your daily fitness fix.

Being flexible in training always works best if you have a specific goal or set of triathlon goals on the horizon to keep you on the right course. So how does being flexible get you to your goal? My best analogy is that of an airplane pilot en route to a destination. A good pilot spends most of the time constantly adjusting the plane's speed, altitude, and direction to get to the destination safely and quickly. All the while, the pilot accounts for unpredictable variables such as changes in wind and weather and factors on the ground, making the appropriate adjustments.

Much like an airplane pilot, the smart triathlete who embraces flexibility has both a flight plan in her head and the wisdom to adjust her training as the need arises. Being flexible assumes you are a self-disciplined and committed person who knows the difference between lactic acid burn and laziness. Here are some tips to help you adopt this more easy-going approach without losing focus:

- Make a plan early in the week for what your training will be like, using the weekly planning format on page 132. Weekly planning is critical.

- Decide what your key workouts will be and how you will incorporate the heart rate and 80/20 training features in chapters 5, 6, and 7. If your schedule is not fixed or is unpredictable, set these workouts as weekly goals and execute them "on the fly." Be self-disciplined, however, in making sure you complete your targeted training by week's end.

- Train with people who have similar goals.

- Pay close attention to injury and overtraining flags and adjust your training accordingly. See page 34 for some common warning signs.

One important note: A flexible schedule may not be for everyone. If you're the type of person who prefers not to deviate at all from your training schedule because the routine helps you to stay focused and on track, then this approach is probably not right for you. Taking on a more flexible scheduling approach is also probably not the best approach for newcomers to the sport. Success in being flexible depends greatly on your proven knowledge of what works and what doesn't work for you (based on previous experience), so you as a rookie triathlete will do better to adhere closely to a proven training plan.

HEALTHY LIFESTYLE

What does a healthier lifestyle have to do with time management? As you get older and more experienced in both life and triathlon, you'll realize that a number of seemingly unrelated lifestyle choices can add up to either some beneficial or detrimental effects on your body. Eventually, those choices work for you or against you as you manage your time. For example, poor nutritional choices eventually affect you in terms of low energy, possibly causing you to be much slower than normal during your long rides and thus throwing off your schedule. Lack of sleep has the same effect on workouts as it does on your overall productivity. Bottom line, your lifestyle choices will have a direct impact on your ability to manage your triathlon training time. In the coming section, we'll cover some of the lifestyle choices that will very likely have an impact on your training, such as nutrition, massage, and other therapies that can help you be a fitter, healthier triathlete.

Tri-Nutrition

Nutrition can be confusing and complex, and new research is rapidly changing the frontiers. In addition, nutrition research is constantly under the watchful eye of the media and is sometimes influenced by corporate sponsors. So things can get complicated, especially when you consider that nutrition and sports nutrition is a multibillion-dollar market for food companies.

You are probably familiar with three nutrients that come from food: carbohydrate, protein, and fat. Each nutrient plays a vital role in the proper functioning of your body, and the ideal amounts of each will help you perform at your best.

Carbohydrate

Most athletes know that carbohydrate is the most important, though least abundant, fuel for energy. The body burns carbohydrate more efficiently than protein or fat. The energy from carbohydrate can be released within exercising muscles up to three times as fast as the energy from fat.

It's generally accepted that the calories in an athlete's diet should be made up of 60 to 70 percent carbohydrate. Rice, pasta, bread, cereal, fruit, dried peas and beans, potatoes, vegetables, and whole-grain breads are examples of foods high in complex carbohydrate. The bulk of the athlete's diet should come from fruits, whole grains, and vegetables.

Protein

The principal role of protein is to build and repair body tissues, including muscles, ligaments, and tendons. This nutrient also plays a part in the production of enzymes and hormones; thus, protein serves a regulatory function. Proteins are composed of individual units called amino acids. There are 20 amino acids, 11 of which the body manufactures. The other nine are essential amino acids that must be ingested in the foods we eat. If you do not consume essential amino acids, your body's ability to produce certain proteins will be impaired, and your health and performance may suffer.

According to recent studies, endurance athletes do appear to need more protein than the average person. However, most Americans eat more protein than they need. To make sure they're balancing their carbohydrate needs with enough protein, endurance athletes should shoot for a 4:1 ratio (Endurance Research Board 2004). The type of exercise you perform may affect amino acid turnover and may dictate protein requirements. Endurance exercise increases amino acid oxidation (breakdown). Resistance exercise enhances protein turnover and muscle synthesis; therefore, both cardiovascular and strength training exercises increase protein requirements for athletes.

Fat

Fat provides a form of stored energy, contributes to healthy skin, and is part of the structure of many hormones and cell membranes. Fat is also a source of fat-soluble vitamins A, D, E, and K. Although there are plenty of low-value saturated fats to choose from, stick to natural (not artificial) animal or vegetable forms of fat. Selecting lean meats and nonfat or low-fat dairy products and limiting butter, margarine, salad dressing, cream sauces, gravies, and fried foods will help you achieve this goal.

Most nutritionists promote a reduction of fat in the American diet—from the current 37 to 40 percent total calories from fat for the average American to fewer than 30 percent, as the new FDA guidelines on food labels recommend. As an athlete or active person, you may even want to consider cutting down fatty foods to around 20 percent of your caloric intake.

Tri-Nutrition on the Run

With a little forethought, you can maintain a good diet that contributes both to your energy level and to your efficiency in training. Your best bet for making sure that you have a good balance of carbohydrate, protein,

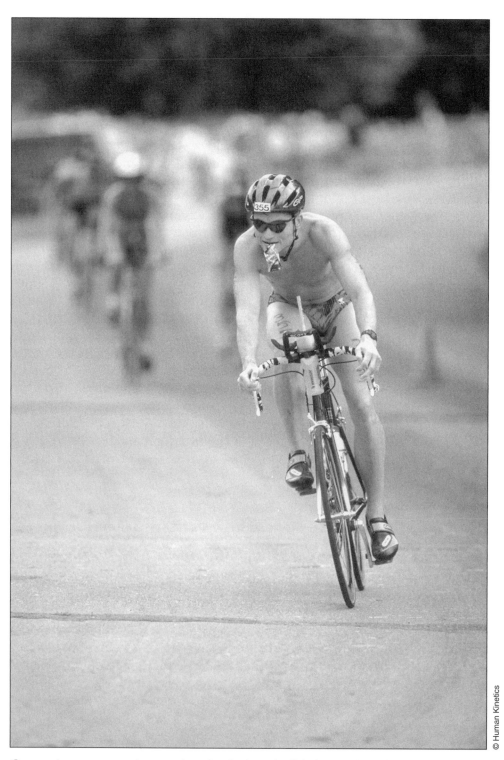

Consuming proper nutrients and staying hydrated will help your body function effectively throughout the race.

© Human Kinetics

and fat in your diet is to keep your pantry stocked with plenty of fruits, vegetables, whole grains, and a variety of other healthy foods. For busy lifestyles that require some nutrition on the go, stick to low-fat grain and fruit snacks such as pretzels, rice cakes, fig bars, and dried fruit. Energy bars that consist of primarily complex carbohydrate, a moderate amount of protein, and little fat are also a good option for the time-strapped.

Tri-Hydration

How much water do you drink during the day? Drinking plenty of water helps your muscles, joints, and other major systems function properly. More than half of your body weight is water, which shows how vital it is. It's especially important to hydrate after training and in the days that follow a particularly demanding workout. For every pound of body weight that you have lost through sweat, you'll need to replace 24 ounces of fluid.

During the times that I have made a real effort to drink plenty of water during the day, my overall energy level has improved and the flexibility in my joints has seemed to increase. It is a healthy lifestyle choice to become a true water drinker, not just on the bike or during a run but constantly during the day. Here are some important facts that may encourage you to keep a water bottle on your desk, in your car, and constantly by your side:

- Your circulatory system is aided by water because water makes up the basis of blood—the higher the content of water in blood, the greater the volume and the more efficiently this system works.
- Water is the basis of the juices in your digestive system, and the greater the amount of fluid along the stomach walls, the easier foods are to digest.
- Water helps keep joints lubricated, because the cartilage that facilitates movement is composed primarily of water.
- An average person loses two to three quarts of water daily from urinating, sweating, and having bowel movements. A triathlete will lose much more because of the higher level of activity.

Most authorities recommend drinking six to eight 8-ounce glasses of water a day. Many factors influence the amount of water you want to consume during the day, most notably the amount of weight you lose through sweat during your workout. You must hydrate regularly—before, during, and after a workout—for recovery and overall health.

Massage Therapy

Taking the time to integrate massage therapy into your lifestyle is another way you can improve your ability to manage time. Granted, on the surface it may seem as though more activities will only fill up your schedule more quickly. However, taking the time to schedule massage therapy will help you recover faster and perform better, with the result of making you more efficient and dialed in to your triathlon training. Whether you schedule a massage once a week or once a month, you'll find the ultimate fitness and performance benefits will far outweigh the hour or two that you invest.

For many years now, professional endurance athletes, such as Tour de France cyclists who must recover quickly between stages, have embraced massage as an integral tool in their training arsenal. That's because working your muscles hard creates microtears in muscle fiber and lactic acid buildup. These conditions can create adhesions, which can manifest themselves in tightness, soreness, and muscle imbalances. Massage can break down these adhesions and flush out toxins, making your muscles prone to quicker recovery.

Massage also has these benefits:

- Strengthens your immune system and improves your body's defenses
- Improves circulation to injured areas and speeds healing
- Makes your muscles and tissues more flexible
- Provides stress relief and relaxation

How often should you get a massage? Ideally, if you are training hard 5 or 6 days a week, you should aim for an hour session once every 1 to 2 weeks with a therapist certified in sport massage. However, if you're strapped for cash or time, aim for once a month at a minimum and supplement your session with self-massage as often as possible.

ENERGY-EFFICIENT EXPENDITURE

Getting the most out of your time will hinge greatly on your ability to smartly expend the limited amount of energy that you have. And there is a limit. Most of us don't think of our own energy (bodily, mental, spiritual) as limited, but if you've ever felt as completely exhausted after you've argued with your spouse as after you've completed a 100-mile bike ride, you know that your limited supply of energy can be depleted in many different ways.

Good time management in triathlon training has as much to do with making wise choices about your energy as it does with your weekly planning grids or your six-month training calendar. Here are some tips for making sure you maximize your energy.

• **Plan easy days around long or intensive workouts.** Certain workouts will obviously take more out of you than others. If you're training for the half-Ironman or Ironman distance, you can count on some long-distance running and cycling that will put a serious crimp in your energy level in the days after your long workouts. Even short interval workouts and other high-energy expenditure training can leave you dragging for a day or two. When doing your weekly planning, schedule an easy workout or day off before your longest distance or your speed work training. Do the same for the day or days afterward, depending on the energy you've expended. Back-to-back killer workouts will only result in burnout and injury.

• **Watch out for post-killer-workout syndrome.** Have you ever felt unusually cranky, fatigued, or short-tempered the day after a 20-mile run or 100-mile bike ride? Of course, your body has been taxed to its limits, and the physical wear and tear are evident. But what you may not be aware of is how the temporary hormonal imbalances and other physiological effects of long-distance or intense exercise can affect your mood, demeanor, and general disposition. I have experienced it many times and have often scratched my head about my behavior and my uncharacteristically sour mood on a Monday, which was usually the off day after my weekend long-distance work on the roadways and running trails. Gradually I came to realize that my mental state was a result of some tough weekend training, and eventually dubbed this phenomenon "post-killer-workout syndrome." Friends and loved ones know to look out for my inner crab and are usually forgiving of my ill-tempered frame of mind.

If your experience is similar, try to plan for post-killer-workout syndrome by not filling your calendar with demanding social events or other activities that may light your short fuse during the day or two following a series of hard training. Delay any demanding obligations or stressful events until your body is more balanced and your mood a little kinder.

• **Plan your workouts at high-energy times.** Sometimes you simply have to train at a given time. Work or family obligations demand you stick to the only time slot left in your day, be it in the morning, during lunchtime, after work, or in the wee hours of night. If possible, however, plan your workouts for the time of day when you know your energy level will be high. Doing so will promote consistent performance, good effort, and solid technique.

• **Plan your workouts to increase energy.** Sometimes the best thing you can do is to take the opposite approach to the previous tip. If an early run or lunchtime swim during your day's lull will energize you to meet the demands of work or family, then that's what works best for you. Self-discipline is critical, however. You need to work out exactly when you probably don't want to. Chances are that once you get out the door or into the swimming pool your energy level will increase. However, be sure to pay attention to maintaining good technique (especially in the pool) if you start out sluggishly.

• **Recognize when not to train.** As we'll discuss in the next chapter, rest is just as important a component of your training schedule as your workouts. In terms of managing your energy, you must also realize there are many different circumstances in which training is not a good idea. Sickness, injury, extreme stress, family crisis, important obligations, and a long list of other reasons unique to your life and circumstances are all grounds for skipping workouts. Recognizing these valid reasons, accepting them, and moving on to the next doable workout are all fundamental steps you need to take in order to keep your energy level consistent throughout your entire training season.

CHAPTER 3

The Master Training Plan

Comfort is a curious thing. We all seek it in one form or another. Yet when we achieve a certain degree of comfort, we may find our lives somewhat limited and even unexciting. Sometimes being in that illusive comfort zone can lead to stagnation and loss of motivation. Challenge is what we all need, whether the challenge is surviving a triathlon swim, hammering the bike, or completing your first Ironman.

Are you in a comfort zone with your triathlon training that is limiting your possibilities? Perhaps a challenge is the springboard you need to propel you out of your rut and into your best triathlon season ever.

Having trained for and finished my first Ironman-distance race, I found that my perception of what I was capable of expanded. The idea of riding more than 100 miles nauseated me at first. But after I completed a 120-mile bike ride and realized I was still standing, subsequent long rides suddenly didn't intimidate me anymore. Having completed this race, I'm starting to consider triathlons and marathons I previously deemed too challenging.

We all tend to pigeonhole ourselves—put ourselves into little boxes with well-defined limitations. As time passes, the walls of these boxes may even get thicker. Sometimes the walls close in on us, and our perception of our own capabilities lessens. If you're mired in the comfort zone and find yourself limited by your own box, entertain the possibility of expanding your horizons as you create your master plan. You don't have to absolutely commit to anything right now. Consider this an exercise in daydreaming. Let a certain challenge or goal—something you've never considered doing before—simmer in your mind. If it sticks around, that probably means it won't go away until you sit down and start creating your master plan.

In this chapter, we'll look at the primary steps and planning strategies you'll need to create a master triathlon training plan. We'll also look at some ways of planning your training so that you stay healthy and avoid being derailed by injury.

TRAINING WEEK GOALS

One of the key tools provided in this book is the weekly planning worksheet on page 132. Doing weekly planning and goal setting is a fundamental concept for triathlon training success (and for achievement in other areas of your life). No matter what period of training you are working in, having goals for each week will keep you focused and on track.

As you review some of the workouts and strive to create your own plan in later chapters, there will obviously be some recurring goals, and some targets will be the same from week to week. The point is that you must commit to a specific goal for the coming week. Here are some tips to help you set your weekly goals.

• **Block off Sunday nights.** Provided you don't have any other important family obligations, Sunday night is usually the ideal time for you to think about and plan your week's goals. Block off 30 minutes to review your training log, look at your training calendar, and consider the goals that you need to focus on in the coming week.

• **Focus on the basic at first.** Your weekly goals should be completely individual. If you are experiencing a lull in motivation and need to focus on something just to get you going, or if you want to overcome a personal weakness that keeps you from training consistently, setting a goal to clear a short-term hurdle is a great idea. For example, maybe you need to get up an hour earlier three times a week to fit in your swimming workout. Until the habit of waking up earlier is ingrained, your goal for the first few weeks of training should be simply to make that happen.

• **Focus on TMG.** As you consider your training goals for the week, think about goals that will do *the most good,* or TMG. Ask yourself a simple question: What can I do this week that will do me the most good for this stage of my triathlon training? This simple question usually leads to the right goal for the week. Such an approach is helpful for setting goals in any endeavor.

BENCHMARKS

Although short-term goals (such as weekly goals) keep you on track and the long-term goal (your race event) is your ultimate motivator, intermediate benchmarks and stepping stones along the way can also prove very helpful. Benchmarks should build on one another, like rungs in a ladder, to lead you up to your ultimate goal.

Benchmarks function as audit checks to ensure that all the work you're doing is taking you where you want to go in your triathlon odyssey. For example, when I was training for my Ironman-distance race, the benchmarks I set were a series of local half-Ironman races that I wanted to complete in a set time (as a middle-of-the-packer, that time was usually under six hours). I also ran additional miles after several of these races to begin preparing mentally to run longer distances at the end of a grueling effort. These races were well-defined measuring sticks for me, and my postrace runs were confidence-building elements that reassured me I had the mental and physical stamina required for the Ironman distance.

Benchmarks differ from long-term goals in that they are strictly progress gauges along the way to achieving your ultimate goal. Whereas your goals may or may not be based on performance, a benchmark must always have some element of measurement, even if it is simply to complete a given workout or race—otherwise, how will you know you've accomplished it? Benchmarks must meet many different criteria in order to be effective targets in your triathlon training program. Here are some guidelines to help you start in the right direction.

• **Space benchmarks apart.** Always schedule your benchmarks within your master training plan so that you have ample time to complete them. Generally speaking, and depending on the length of your training schedule, always set these miniachievements several months apart—although you may find that a majority of them are appropriately set for the latter part of your season. Make sure you mark and circle them on your training calendar as a visual cue. Use table 12.2 on page 131 to help you brainstorm and document your benchmarks.

• **Make benchmarks meaningful.** Benchmarks should be significant indicators that you are making steady progress toward your long-term goal. You may only have two or three benchmarks within your master plan. Don't make them trivial or minor—give them appropriate weight and importance by setting a challenging bar to reach.

• **Make benchmarks measurable.** Whether it's a particular race or a training course time, each benchmark should be somehow measurable. The measure can be simply finishing a 20-mile run, a 60-mile bike ride, or a mile in the swimming pool without stopping. Going for either a set time or mere completion ensures you have a way of measuring your success.

PRECAUTIONS AGAINST INJURY

The biggest key to avoiding injury is really quite simple in concept but much, much harder in execution—high adaptability. What does it mean? Adaptability means that at every stage of your triathlon odyssey, from planning to training to racing, you must be receptive to your body's signals in order to make quick and timely adjustments.

When setting up your training plan, it's vital to plan and execute your training defensively. You've all heard the term that the safest drivers drive defensively, with a vigilant mindset and the wherewithal to recognize dangerous behavior. If you want to safeguard your body and avoid injury, planning your triathlon training with the same kind of defensive mindset is the single best thing you can do for yourself.

As you sit down to plan your schedule, listen for those instincts that may be telling you you're overloading yourself or stacking too many workouts on top of each other, which may break down your body. Besides listening to your gut, you can use the following tips for planning your training defensively:

• **Plan your running carefully.** Unless you are one of the few triathletes blessed with the perfect runner's body, flawless form, and near-perfect technique, pounding the pavement is the activity (of the three disciplines) with the highest probability of injury. A five-year study by Staffordshire University of 116 triathletes with differing abilities—from elite triathlete to weekend warrior—showed that 58 to 64 percent of all overuse injuries stemmed from running (Vleck and Garbutt 1998). Be very careful when increasing distance or intensity abruptly, without giving your body a chance to adapt. Always plan an easy workout after a high-intensity or long run and never increase your total weekly running distance by more than 10 percent from week to week.

• **Lean toward safety.** There may be several critical points in your training at which you feel a certain workout may be pushing it or that your body's ability to safely finish that extra long run or that unusually hilly bike ride is suspect. Although some measure of risk is acceptable, there's no shame in playing it safe by reducing the intensity or distance (or both) of these demanding workouts. If your gut tells you that you may be skirting that fine line between better performance and injury, err on the side of caution and make the necessary training adjustments. As you sit down to plan or review upcoming training, shave off some distance, notch down the intensity, or consider an easier course if you feel that your body may be on the brink of overuse.

• **Avoid the superman syndrome.** Anybody who has ever had a sports injury can probably point to a specific workout or a series of efforts over a short period of time that caused it. Unless injury is caused by something traumatic—a fall on the bike, a dog bite on a run—the root cause is usually overuse that can be clearly mapped in a training log. So if it's so easy to document an injury afterward, why is it so hard to avoid one? Part of the answer is that we become so attached to our training that our self-image and ego become entangled in it, making it hard to accept the blatantly obvious warning signs. This so-called superman mentality can fool you into believing one more track workout or one extra set of ascending laps will do no harm. That's why reviewing your daily training log entries from the previous weeks and months on a consistent basis is so important—it keeps you in tune with the reality of your recent training. Examining

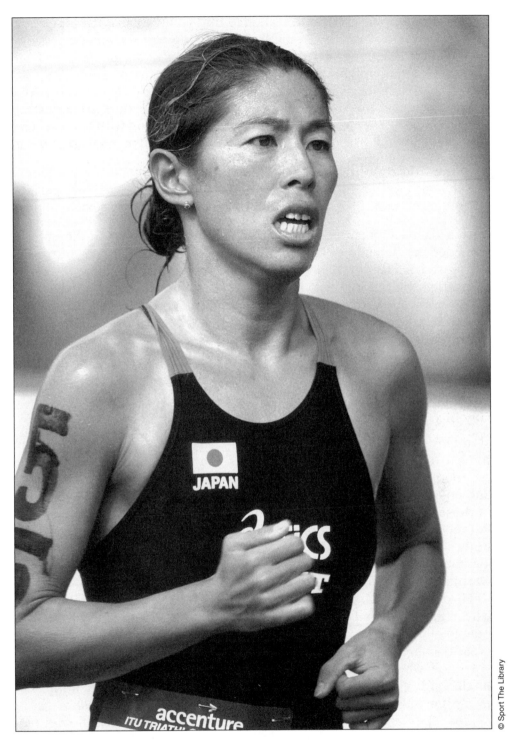

Planning your running carefully will help you avoid overuse injuries and will put you on the road to the finish line.

your log can provide valuable evidence that an injury may be imminent, giving you an opportunity to dial down training and allow your body an opportunity to recover from any cumulative muscle tissue damage from several weeks of tough workouts.

During demanding peak training periods, make some time to take a deep breath (literally), step back, and examine your training with an objective eye. Doing so can help you to better see warning signs so that you can adjust your training to avoid injury.

REST DAYS

Rest is just as important as training. Is that hard for you to swallow? If so, consider the benefits of training that actually materialize in your body with rest. It's a fact that endurance sports are very stressful on the body. Every time we put in a hard run, climb hills on our bikes, and swim lap after lap, we stress our muscles, ligaments, and tendons. On a physiological level, cells are damaged through tears on the membranes. This means that putting in the miles and meters delivers a pretty good wallop to our bodies. It's during our posttraining recovery time that these microtears heal, which ultimately makes our muscles stronger.

The stress of overtraining affects a number of organs and systems in your body, causing a ripple effect that manifests itself in many symptoms. Since everyone's body is unique, symptoms of overtraining will vary substantially from triathlete to triathlete. Some possible overtraining symptoms to look out for are pain in the joints, crankiness and a general feeling of moodiness, eye sensitivity to light, fatigue, insomnia, poor digestion, and an inability to elevate heart rate properly. If you find one or several of these symptoms plaguing you, then it's time to throttle back and give yourself a few more days of rest. These are just a few examples of the body's potential reaction to stress; however, you may have noticed some symptoms that are unique to you. Learn to listen to your body when the warning flags are hoisted and back off on your training.

Through the years, triathletes have found that interspersing training with rest has helped improve both the odds of avoiding injury and the quality of performance. The core training concept embodied by triathlon, cross-training, is in itself a tool for helping the body to recover. But how do you know when you're pushing your limits; where is that elusive redline on the body's injury-o-meter? There's no clear-cut answer that applies to everyone, but there are steps you can take to minimize the risk.

Most sport injuries are a result of not allowing the body enough rest and recovery time. Planning and following a smart and effective training schedule that builds in rest days and easy training or cross-training days for recovery are crucial to avoiding injury. The challenge is that many triathletes have a difficult time resting. Triathlon training can become an addiction, sometimes to the point of being unhealthy. To counter this tendency, make a commitment to stick to a training schedule that builds in some days with little or no activity so that your body can recover. As mentioned previously, you should plan these days immediately after what you know will be a long or tough workout. For example, I do most of my long runs on Sunday mornings, so on Mondays I usually either rest completely or go for an easy swim.

Take your rest days as seriously as you take your training days. You may also want to schedule a massage or some other relaxing activity on your rest days. In the long run, nurturing your body on these days off will help you be more productive and efficient on training days.

TAPERING

Tapering in training is a decrease of distance, intensity, or a combination of both in the days or weeks before a race. Although tapering may be my favorite training cycle, for many die-hard triathletes that have become addicted to the adrenaline rush of training it may well be the least favorite. I suppose it's all in the attitude. I look at tapering as a time to take the intensity of training down a notch—even take a few days off—and sit back and reflect on all the hard work I've done to become a tri-fit athlete. I also take time to devote myself to mentally preparing for the big event. Whether you find it rejuvenating or frustrating, tapering works. Studies have proven that decreasing exercise intensity, volume, or both before a race helps the body recover in time for a peak performance.

In a study at Malaspina College in British Columbia and the University of Alberta there was a 12 percent increase of the lactate threshold level in athletes who tapered for as little as three days (Neary et al. 1992). The lactate threshold is a measure of how long a certain exercise intensity can be maintained. The higher the threshold, the greater your ability to sustain exercise at a high level. (The actual burning sensation in your quads when you climb a hill is called lactic acid burn, which happens as soon as your body crosses that threshold during sustained, high-intensity exercise.)Those in the study that trained up until race day showed a decrease in their lactate threshold. But take heed—those in the aforementioned study who did absolutely no exercise for a full week before race day also showed a decrease in their lactate threshold, although it was not as significant as in the overtrained group. The lesson we learn from this study is that tapering should be a metaphoric easing of the foot on the gas pedal or a downshift into a lower gear, not an abrupt braking that causes you to lose some of your physical and mental edge. When you create your training schedule, planning a tapering program before your races will ensure that you are fresh and race ready at the starting line. In the training programs in chapters 8 through 11, you'll also find specific tapering recommendations based on your race distance goal.

PLANNING AN EIGHT-WEEK WORKOUT MATRIX

In part III, you'll find chapters divided into the four major triathlon race distances. Each contains tables that show eight-week training matrices, or what I like to call snapshots of what training may entail in the months leading up to a race. As you sit down to plan your training season, refer to these tables. These snapshots are your starting point for creating a customized plan that is appropriate for your current fitness and ability level and is aligned with the relevant phase of your season calendar. Of course, training in most distances will require more than an eight-week effort. As you create your master plan and divide your training calendar into blocks of weeks and months, use the goals and benchmarks that you've created to help sharpen your focus and energize your training. Doing so lays the groundwork for refining your training plan in the upcoming chapters.

PART II

Customized Training

You are unique, and your training should reflect your uniqueness. That's why this section provides a generous sampling of many different types of workouts and training considerations. From finding your heart rate zones to fitting in a workout during your lunch hour to doing a perfect brick, you'll find here the information you need to start planning workouts that will help you manage your valuable time, meet your goals, and get you to the finish line feeling strong.

CHAPTER 4

Heart Rate Workouts

One of my fondest memories is of a very tough Fourth of July 10K race in Lemont, a western suburb of Chicago best known for the Cog Hill golf course and very hilly roads (relatively speaking, for the Midwest). I'd just purchased a heart rate monitor and programmed it to beep when my heart rate fell above or below my target range. As anyone who has run a hilly road race knows, it's tough to maintain a steady pace, let alone a steady heart rate.

But I held back when my heart rate told me to in the first few miles and pushed when it told me to in the last few miles. I managed to stay in the target range most of the time and came close to a personal record (PR) on a very hilly course. Best of all, I beat a longtime rival who usually smoked me.

Heart rate training can be one of the most valuable tools in your training arsenal, giving you valuable input from your body that you can use to train more efficiently and plan future workouts more effectively. In this chapter we'll take you through the fundamentals of heart rate training, including some sample workouts. Since heart rate training is so integral to an efficient training plan, you'll also find several workouts in upcoming chapters that use the principles discussed here.

HEART RATE PRIMER

Triathlon training is all about intensity. How hard should you swim, bike, and run? It's a question that every triathlete asks before donning the swimsuit, bike shorts, or running shoes. Heart rate training is designed to answer that question with a degree of accuracy that only today's high-tech monitors can give you. By knowing your heart rate and the right zones you should be training in during any given workout, you'll be in sync with your body and current fitness level, which will help you plan each workout with your goals firmly within reach.

To determine exactly how you will use heart rate training in your program, you first need to determine a couple of different factors that are unique to you, such as your maximum heart rate and your resting heart rate. Once you have determined what those are by using the Karvonen formula, you'll be able to determine the heart rate zones that you should be staying within during each workout.

DETERMINING YOUR ZONES

You may be familiar with the heart rate formula that simply subtracts your age from 220 to determine your maximum heart rate and subsequent target zones, based on that number. The Karvonen formula, however, factors in an element important for helping you determine a more precise method of training—resting heart rate. This formula factors in both age and average resting heart rate to accurately determine your level of fitness conditioning. Although there are other methods of calculating, we'll be using the Karvonen formula for the purposes of this text.

Figure 4.1, at the end of the chapter, will help you determine your heart rate zones using the method described in the following sections. You'll also be able to make sport-specific adjustments, among others.

Average Resting Heart Rate

Your resting heart rate is best determined when you first awake in the morning. If you usually wake in a stressful manner, such as to a blaring alarm clock radio or the kids jumping on your stomach, try starting your day in a calmer way for at least three days in a row. For example, recruit your spouse to gently wake you with a pleasant voice or touch, or try one of the new light, soft chime, or low-vibrating alarms that are less shocking to your system. While you're still in bed and in a restful state, use a watch to count your heart beats per minute. Do this every morning for three days, and then calculate your average resting heart rate. To get an average, add your three resting rate numbers together and divide by three. This number is a good indicator of your current level of conditioning: The fitter you are, the lower your resting heart rate, which means your heart is pumping more efficiently with fewer beats per minute.

Please note, however, that you should always take your resting heart rate on days when your exercise regime is normal and your body is relatively well rested, not after high-intensity track intervals or a 20-mile run. Your resting heart rate will very likely be higher than normal on days after such hard efforts.

Target Zones

Target training zones are a range of heart rates designed for a specific purpose. Training in zones gives you a clear purpose and direction for your workouts, giving you the confidence that you're working toward your goal smartly and efficiently.

Determining your heart rate training zones helps you plan your swimming, biking, and running workouts to achieve specific results, such as raising your lactate threshold. As you create your training schedule, you'll be using heart rate zones to design your individual workout to achieve the results you need for each phase of your seasonal training calendar.

Athletes use several different ways to delineate target zones, and some experts divide targets into as many as five zones. To help streamline your training, this book covers three primary target zones: the recovery and endurance zone, the aerobic and tempo zone, and the anaerobic threshold zone. As you become more sophisticated and detailed in working with heart rate training, you may opt to structure your training with as many as five target zones.

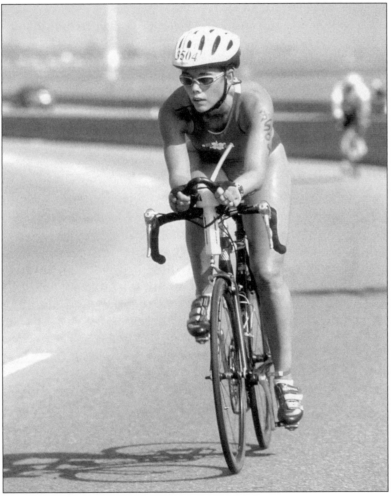

© Dennis Light

Heart rate training helps you get in—and stay in—your target zone during your race.

To determine your zones, begin by subtracting your age from 220 (this gives you your estimated maximum heart rate). From this number, subtract your average resting heart rate. This is your zone baseline number, which is important in calculating your individual zones.

Recovery and Endurance Zone (60-70%)

This training zone is the best for recovery workouts. When you've had a long or high-intensity workout that has really pushed your limits, this zone helps you consolidate the benefits from your hard work with an easy effort that gives your body a chance to rejuvenate. It is also the zone to work in when building your endurance base, as when you do a long, slow distance run to help lay a good fitness foundation early on in a training season. Training in this zone to build your endurance gives you the benefit of safely increasing your fitness incrementally while giving your body a chance to adapt to increasing distances. It also lays a solid groundwork for higher-intensity training down the road.

To determine the lower limit of your recovery and endurance zone, multiply your baseline number by the zone multiplier .60 (60%). Add your average resting heart rate to this number. The resulting number is the lower heart rate limit of your recovery and endurance zone.

To determine the upper limit of your recovery and endurance zone, multiply your baseline number by the zone multiplier .70 (70%). Add your average resting heart rate to this number. The number you get is the upper heart rate limit of your recovery and endurance zone.

Aerobic and Tempo Zone (70-80%)

This zone reflects a higher intensity that results in a greater degree of aerobic power, an improvement often known as the training effect. Improving your aerobic power means that your respiratory system becomes more efficient, advancing your body's ability to transport oxygen to muscles while simultaneously expelling carbon dioxide away from muscles. Training in the aerobic and tempo zone builds on your fitness foundation and—over a period of time—makes you strong enough to swim, run, and bike for longer periods and at greater speed. Once you've established your base foundation, you will do the majority of your training in this zone.

To determine your lower and upper limits for the aerobic and tempo zone, take the same formula I described for the recovery zone, but use the lower and upper zone multipliers of .70 and .80, respectively.

Anaerobic Threshold Zone (80-90%)

This zone represents the highest intensity workout that you would typically experience during a track interval workout or during a tough climb on your road bike. Your anaerobic threshold is the point at which you go from an aerobic to anaerobic state. You will very likely feel a burning sensation in your legs during a steep climb on your bike, for example, because the lactic acid in your leg muscles accumulates faster than your body can remove it. The anaerobic threshold zone represents a level of high-intensity training that you should reserve for interval workouts on the track or other demanding sessions. You should strategically bookend these workouts with easy recovery workouts to avoid overtraining and to keep yourself mentally and physically fresh. Though difficult in nature, training in this zone reaps tremendous benefits in speed and stamina. Working in this zone can also help your technique and form in all three sports, provided you consciously focus on maintaining proper form under the pressure of these workouts.

To determine your anaerobic threshold zone, use the zone multipliers of .80 and .90 for your lower and upper limits, respectively.

ZONE ADJUSTMENTS

Once you know your target zones, you must still do a little tweaking of the range numbers in order to further individualize your training for improved accuracy and efficiency. All training has to be individualized, and these adjustments take into account the different characteristics of each sport, outside conditions, and any illness or overtraining symptoms that may be happening within your body.

Some adjustments are sport-specific. It's become obvious to me through the years that my heart rate while running is at least 10 beats higher than a similar perceived effort while riding my bike. That's not uncommon, since running puts a pretty good wallop on the legs and causes a greater degree of stress on major muscle groups from the impact. Cycling is less stressful on joints, often resulting in a lower heart rate, and swimming is even less taxing.

To adjust for the unique demands of all three sports, you may want to adjust your training zones for cycling to be 10 fewer beats than what you would use for running. For example, if you've field-tested the target zone numbers you derived with the given formulas on a few runs at various intensities, then subtract 10 beats from your lower and upper limits in each zone to determine your cycling zones. For swimming, adjust your target zones down 5 beats from your adjusted cycling target zones.

You would also be wise to make a number of other adjustments to your heart rate training, depending on altitude, weather, and illness.

• **Altitude adjustments.** If you are training or traveling to a race above an altitude of 6,000 feet (1,830 meters) for the first time, or if you do so infrequently, your heart rate will naturally be higher, even at rest. Above 10,000 feet (3,050 meters), you may find your heart rate is a full 50 percent higher. This increase is due to the lower concentration of oxygen in the air at higher altitudes. Of course, the more time you spend at higher altitudes, the greater your body's ability to adapt, and you'll probably see a return to your normal heart rate levels after 14 to 21 days. In fact, you can track your acclimatization with your heart rate monitor, noting how your rate decreases and finally gets back to normal within a few weeks. During this time of acclimatization, don't push beyond your ability, and stay in your target zones. This means that you may have to slow down or lower the intensity of your training in the interim. Be patient—your body will adjust.

• **Hot-weather adjustments.** Exercising in hot weather causes your body to work harder to keep itself cool. Increased blood flow to the skin and sweating cause an elevated heart rate response. The good news is that consistent training in heat brings about acclimatization in much the same way altitude training does. The body becomes much more efficient in dealing with the heat, resulting in a normal blood flow, decreased salt content in sweat, and a return to your normal heart rate. This adjustment usually takes about 10 days of consistent training or about half a dozen workouts in hot conditions. Always remember to hydrate properly (in hot or cold weather, but it's usually more critical in heat). Dehydration can decrease your total blood volume, making the heart work harder and elevating your heart rate.

• **Illness.** If you find that your resting heart rate has spiked unusually or that it is more difficult than normal to reach your target zones, it may well be that you are courting an illness such as a cold or flu. If you experience either or both of these conditions, back off and take a rest day or a few easy recovery workouts.

THE OVERTRAINING ZONE

Difficulty getting your heart rate to its normal level during a workout is an indicator that you may be overtraining. This is another reason heart rate training can be beneficial—it provides a link between you and your body that teaches you to become more attuned to what is happening. If you fail to listen to your body and your heart rate monitor, the inability to get into your training zone may lead to further overtraining. The failure of blood vessels to constrict, due to cortisol depletion caused by overtraining, lowers the peak heart rate threshold. A heart rate monitor may prove deceptive in such a case; although the monitor may imply you're not pushing hard enough because your heart rate is lower than normal, you may already have pushed too hard. Discerning the fine line between high-performance training and overdoing is a constant challenge, even for professional athletes who earn their keep from racing triathlons. Your training logs should be your most valuable tool when you suspect you are pushing that line. By objectively reviewing your last few weeks' worth of training, you should be able to spot clues and patterns of overtraining.

Another indication of overtraining is your body's inability to recover between repeats during an interval workout. You should generally be able to recover to a normal heart rate after about 120 beats, although it's not an exact measurement. You should first determine what your normal individual recovery rate is. Of course, your fitness level also influences your ability to recover. If you've established a normal recovery rate over a period of time and find yourself taking longer to recover between intervals, then chances are it's time to get off the track and take a day or two off.

HEART RATE WORKOUTS

Heart rate training is a valuable tool that you can apply to any type of workout. In fact, it is most useful when you have a very specific goal or focus in your training, which is why heart rate recommendations are integrated with many of the forthcoming workouts in the following three chapters, as well as with the distance-specific training grids in part III of this book.

To get you started right away, here are three sample heart rate workouts in several distances with suggested modifications to apply to any race. As you'll see, there are many creative ways to use heart rate monitoring to make training fun while boosting your performance and training efficiency.

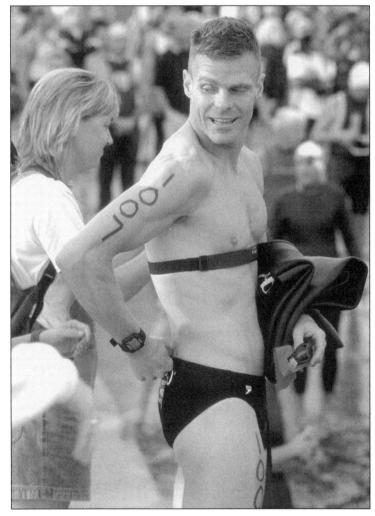

Forget about the funky tan lines. Wearing a heart rate monitor during the race will contribute to a peak performance.

© Human Kinetics

▶ *FAST RECOVERY SWIM WORKOUT (SPRINT DISTANCE)*

Swimming with a heart rate monitor can be problematic if you depend on the zone alarm feature, which chimes when you hit the lower or upper limits of your specified range. It may be difficult to hear the chime while swimming and nearly impossible if you wear ear plugs. If this is the case for you, a workout that uses the heart rate monitor as a tool for measuring and improving your ability to recover between intervals is a good solution. Such a workout will not only increase your overall fitness, it will help you to recover and perform better during the inevitable peaks and valleys of racing.

Warm-up: Swim at an easy pace for up to 10 minutes, starting slowly and gradually raising your heart rate to your recovery and endurance zone. It's OK to stop for a few seconds between laps to check your heart rate if you have trouble hearing the chime.

Workout: Swim a series of 6 intervals of 50 meters each at high intensity, aiming for your heart rate to rise rapidly into the anaerobic threshold zone. Rest between intervals until your heart rate falls into the recovery and endurance zone, then begin the next 50 meters. It may take several intervals before your heart rate reaches the anaerobic threshold zone, especially if you're particularly fit; if this is the case, increase your high-intensity interval distance to 75 or 100 meters.

Distance modifications: Modify for longer races by increasing the number of intervals by 2 for each triathlon distance (8 for Olympic, 10 for half-Ironman, 12 for Ironman).

Cool-down: Swim at an easy pace for 10 minutes, preferably throwing in a few technique drills.

▶ *CYCLING CRISSCROSS WORKOUT (SPRINT OR OLYMPIC DISTANCE)*

The crisscross is a great workout that helps you become more in tune with how subtle changes in your exertion can affect your heart rate during a race. It also fosters a feeling of mastery and control of your body—a valuable confidence-boosting advantage you can carry into any race. This workout should be performed on a flat course or on a trainer.

Warm-up: Cycle at an easy pace for up to 15 minutes, gradually raising your heart rate from your recovery and endurance zone to your aerobic and tempo zone.

Workout: Once in your aerobic and tempo zone, increase your exertion to reach the upper limit of the zone until your alarm chimes. Gradually decrease your exertion until the lower-limit chime kicks in. Increase your exertion until the upper-limit chime sounds. Continue this pattern of crisscrossing the zone for 20 to 30 minutes. If your heart rate were charted on a graph, you would see a consistent peak and valley pattern framed by your aerobic and tempo zone limits.

Distance modifications: For half-Ironman racing, increase your crisscross session to 30 to 40 minutes. For an Ironman, increase to 40 to 50 minutes. As you extend the distance and time, this pattern becomes a more mentally challenging task to execute. If you need it, give yourself a 5- to 10-minute break from crisscrossing in the middle of the workout.

Cool-down: Ride for 10 to 15 minutes, doing easy recovery spinning in your recovery and endurance zone.

▶ *RUNNING LADDERS (HALF-IRONMAN)*

Contrary to what it sounds like, this ladder exercise is not a hilly workout but one that raises the tempo of a run by targeting higher and higher heart rate increments (or rungs in a ladder), and then allows for gradual recovery as you work your way down the ladder (sometimes these workouts are also known as pyramids). This regimen can be considered a type of high-intensity workout and will improve your stamina, leg strength, and running efficiency.

Warm-up: Run at an easy pace for 15 minutes, gradually raising your heart rate during the last 5 minutes to your recovery and endurance zone.

Workout: Set your watch or heart rate monitor to beep every 5 minutes and begin the countdown after your warm-up. Run the first 5 minutes within the bottom 5-beat range of your recovery and endurance zone. Run each subsequent 5-minute segment at a heart rate that is 5 beats faster, until you've done six 5-minute increments (but do not exceed your anaerobic threshold zone). Then begin decreasing 5 beats every 5 minutes, until you've reached the bottom of your recovery and endurance zone once more.

Distance modifications: You can decrease this 60-minute run for sprint- or Olympic-distance training by shortening it to increments of 2 to 4 ascending and 2 to 4 descending rungs. For Ironman training, increase to eight 5-minute increments, but do not exceed the upper limit of your anaerobic threshold zone.

Cool-down: Run at an easy pace or walk for 10 minutes.

Figure 4.1   Heart Rate Worksheet

Step 1: Determine Your Average Resting Heart Rate (HR)

	Resting heart rate
Day 1	
Day 2	
Day 3	
Add your resting heart rates.	
Divide by 3 to determine your resting heart rate.	

Step 2: Determine Your HR Baseline

1. 220 – _____ (age) = _____ (maximum HR)

2. _____ (maximum HR) – _____ (average resting HR) = _____ zone baseline

Step 3: Calculate Your Target Zones

Recovery and Endurance Zone (60-70%)

_____ (zone baseline) x .60 = _____ + _____ (resting HR) = _____ (lower limit)

_____ (zone baseline) x .70 = _____ + _____ (resting HR) = _____ (upper limit)

Your recovery and endurance zone: _____ to _____

Aerobic and Tempo Zone (70-80%)

_____ (zone baseline) x .70 = _____ + _____ (resting HR) = _____ (lower limit)

_____ (zone baseline) x .80 = _____ + _____ (resting HR) = _____ (upper limit)

Your aerobic and tempo zone: _____ to _____

Anaerobic Threshold Zone (80-90%)

_____ (zone baseline) x .80 = _____ + _____ (resting HR) = _____ (lower limit)

_____ (zone baseline) x .90 = _____ + _____ (resting HR) = _____ (upper limit)

Your anaerobic threshold zone: _____ to _____

Step 4: Make Sport-Specific Adjustments

Cycling Target Zones—Use the target zones you've calculated above:

Recovery and endurance:

_____ (upper range) – 10 = _____ (adjusted upper range)

_____ (lower range) – 10 = _____ (adjusted lower range)

Your cycling recovery and endurance zone: _____ to _____

Aerobic and tempo:

_____ (upper range) – 10 = _____ (adjusted upper range)

_____ (lower range) – 10 = _____ (adjusted lower range)

Your cycling aerobic and tempo zone: _____ to _____

Anaerobic threshold:

_____ (upper range) – 10 = _____ (adjusted upper range)

_____ (lower range) – 10 = _____ (adjusted lower range)

Your cycling anaerobic threshold zone: _____ to _____

Swimming Target Zones—Use the target zones you've calculated above:

Recovery and endurance:

_____ (upper range) – 5 = _____ (adjusted upper range)

_____ (lower range) – 5 = _____ (adjusted lower range)

Your swimming recovery and endurance zone: _____ to _____

Aerobic and tempo:

_____ (upper range) – 5 = _____ (adjusted upper range)

_____ (lower range) – 5 = _____ (adjusted lower range)

Your swimming aerobic and tempo zone: _____ to _____

Anaerobic threshold:

_____ (upper range) – 5 = _____ (adjusted upper range)

_____ (lower range) – 5 = _____ (adjusted lower range)

Your swimming anaerobic threshold zone: _____ to _____

Step 5: Make Other Adjustments

Make any additional adjustments for these conditions:

- Altitude
- Hot weather
- Illness
- Any other conditions that might affect heart rate: _____
  _____

CHAPTER 5

Time-Based Workouts

The greatest obstacle to training consistently for your triathlon goal will probably not be the terrain, the elements, or even an injury. More than likely, time will be the limiting factor. Like most things in life, success in triathlon training is directly proportionate to your ability to fit it in during the course of a busy day. Given the requirements of your career, marriage, kids, and lawn, finding time to train can be a real conundrum. In fact, the concept of *finding time* is part of the problem. The distinction between *finding time* and *making time* may seem to be small, but it is really as vast as an Ironman course.

You may never find the time to train if you have a thriving career and a busy family life. There will always be something that has to get done or a spouse or child that needs attention, and rightly so. But when you make time by purposefully apportioning a time slot in your schedule or creating more time (e.g., by working out during your lunch hour) and by rearranging your obligations so that your training can happen consistently, then you've mastered triathlon time management.

This chapter focuses on different time-based workouts, based on different times of day or days of the week, with recommendations on how to get the most out of them. These scenarios may already be playing out in your life, but you may find one or more workouts that will help you squeeze a little more into your busy lifestyle.

MORNING WORKOUTS

We've all heard the term *morning person*. Although it's true that some of us are definitely predisposed to sleeping late, being at peak form early in the day is largely a matter of habit. Morning workouts are usually the best option for individuals faced with a hectic schedule that leaves little wiggle room. Getting up an hour or more earlier requires a commitment of energy and dedication that may be difficult at first, but the rewards are well worth it. Eventually, your morning training session may become your favorite time of day.

Mornings are an ideal time to train for several reasons:

- Exercise jump-starts the day with a heart-pounding activity that isn't the result of that morning cup of coffee.
- Exercise clears the mind and allows you an opportunity to gather your thoughts, amply preparing you for the challenging day ahead.
- Facing the elements—whether the cold slap of water in a swimming pool or the crisp air of a fall run—can invigorate and motivate you for the rest of the day.
- Exercising early clears your schedule for other important obligations.
- Exercising early eliminates any uncertainty about somehow fitting in a workout during the rest of the day.
- Early exercise doesn't conflict with family responsibilities (provided your morning workouts are the result of rising earlier).

Preparation

Preparation is the key to a successful morning workout routine; the easier you can make it on yourself (especially if you don't consider yourself a morning person) the greater your chances of success. As with any activity you wish to make a habit, you want it to be automatic, so the less you have to think about your clothes, your schedule, and making it to work on time, the better.

If you're going to change your sleeping habits and wake earlier, gradually get to bed earlier so that your body can slowly adjust to the new schedule. Prepare your swimming, cycling, and running gear the evening or night before—have you clothes laid out and a gym bag ready next to your bed if you'll be swimming. Don't forget to make sure your bike tires are properly inflated and your gear is ready for a bike ride.

Sample Morning Workouts

Just about any workout can be done in the morning—the real constraint is time. Whatever you decide to do in the morning, make sure you give yourself sufficient time to warm up and ease into the activity, especially if you'll be pounding the pavement or rolling down the roads within minutes of jumping out of bed. We've discussed some of the advantages of early morning workouts, but an additional benefit worth mentioning is you become accustomed to getting the heart pounding early, as virtually all races entail. Since most triathlon race starts closely follow dawn, having a good mental attitude and energy level that has been cultivated by consistent early morning workouts gives you a decisive edge over the competition. Following is a sampling of morning training workouts in various distances to consider.

▶ *MORNING SWIM WORKOUT (SPRINT DISTANCE)*

This workout provides an excellent opportunity to build stamina in as little time as possible. By sustaining a steady pace over a moderate distance, you'll also improve your endurance in the water.

Warm-up: 75 meters easy

Workout: 700 meters at a steady, sustainable, nonstop pace

Cool-down: 50 meters easy

▶ *MORNING BIKE WORKOUT (OLYMPIC DISTANCE)*

Spinning at moderately high revolutions per minute (RPM) is a great way to improve your pedaling technique and efficiency. It's also a great base-building workout that helps you avoid cycling injuries down the road. You'll need a bike computer with a cadence feature.

Warm-up: 5 minutes at an easy pace

Workout: 15 miles (24 kilometers) of easy spinning at 90 RPM or higher

Cool-down: 5 minutes in an easy gear, followed by getting up off the saddle to stretch your hamstrings and legs

▶ *MORNING RUN WORKOUT (IRONMAN DISTANCE)*

The first minutes or miles (or kilometers) of a morning run are always the hardest, so cut yourself some slack and ease into it. This session is ideal for recovery from a hard or long workout, since it gives you an opportunity to consolidate your body's efforts.

Warm-up: Walk for 5 minutes or run the first 5 minutes of the workout very slowly.

Workout: Run for 60 minutes at an easy pace. Feel free to throw in a burst of speed in the middle of the workout to get the adrenaline going.

Cool-down: Walk for 5 minutes or run the last 5 minutes of your workout very slowly.

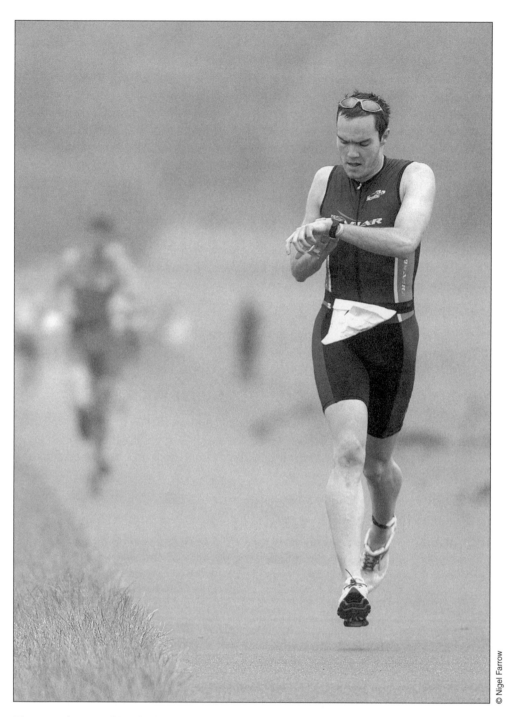

Time can be your friend—during both training and racing—if you manage it properly.

LUNCHTIME WORKOUTS

If your schedule is so squeezed that something's got to give in order for you to get that workout in during your work week, there's no better solution than the good old lunchtime workout. For desk jockeys and cubicle dwellers, the lunch hour can be precious time to get in a decent workout, provided you have the resources (such as a nearby pool or health club, a running or cycling route near your workplace, and shower facilities) to pull it off. Of course, you still want to make sure you get all the proper nutrients, as discussed in chapter 2, so make sure to have a quick, high-nutrition snack or nutritious energy bar after your workout.

Training during your lunch hour has many advantages:

- It gives you an hour to train without throwing off your schedule for the rest of the day.
- It can energize you and help you bypass the typical energy drain of an office environment in the afternoons; it can actually make you more productive at work.
- It allows you an opportunity to get a midday break from your work routine.
- If you have co-workers who train during lunch, it gives you an opportunity to bond and cultivate a positive and healthy fitness culture at work.
- It may encourage your employer to provide health club facilities and showers as an added benefit.

Preparation

Fitting in a lunchtime workout while also keeping your career and work obligations humming can be a real tough juggling act. If your workday excursions cut into your productivity, your employer may not encourage them. Every situation is unique—people who have more freedom and flexibility at work (the boss, telecommuters) are in a much better position to go for a quick bike ride or a fast trip to the YMCA pool. The key is to take a look at your situation and determine what is the most seamless, unobtrusive, and nonthreatening (to your job security) workout strategy for you.

Discussing your lunchtime workout plan with your employer or human resource manager is also important, especially if you suspect your training will affect your availability (such as if you're always on call) or have any impact on the schedules of colleagues. Although there's no guarantee, most employers will appreciate your forthrightness and your commitment to both your profession and fitness.

For a lunchtime workout, preparation is the key—do you have all the gear and shower toiletries to pull it off? Be prepared with plan B if work circumstances make it difficult or impossible to get away to train during your lunch hour. Also, make sure you allot enough time to shower and get back to work on time.

Sample Lunchtime Workouts

Because of the short amount of time available for lunchtime workouts (when you factor in changing, showering, and travel time to where you're training) you should exercise at an intensity that is moderate to high; you won't be able to get in much distance in 30 to 45 minutes, but you can still get in a good hard workout that will definitely contribute to your master plan. During a higher-intensity, shorter workout you'll very likely be approaching your lactate threshold, so training at this level will condition your body to work more efficiently.

▶ *LUNCHTIME SWIM WORKOUT (HALF-IRONMAN)*

Here's a workout that combines the efficiency gains that come from working on technique with the speed improvements that come from swimming at a fast pace.

Warm-up: 50 meters easy

Workout: 4 × 75 meters at a fast, almost unsustainable speed; 2 × 75 meters very easy, focusing on technique; and 4 × 75 meters at a fast, almost unsustainable speed, all with 20 to 30 seconds rest between each 75-meter interval

Cool-down: 50 meters easy

▶ *LUNCHTIME BIKE WORKOUT (SPRINT DISTANCE)*

A heart rate monitor will ensure that you meet your target zones.

Warm-up: 5 minutes spinning in an easy gear

Workout: 5 to 7 miles (8 to 11 kilometers) in aerobic and tempo zone with three 1-minute bursts, sprints, or hill climbs that take you to the top of the zone or slightly above

Cool-down: 5 minutes in an easy gear, then stretching your hamstrings and legs

▶ *LUNCHTIME RUN WORKOUT (OLYMPIC DISTANCE)*

Again, you should focus on a moderate- to high-intensity workout that makes the best use of limited time. *Fartlek* (speed play) can do this for you. Fartlek running is any spontaneous, high-intensity burst in the middle of a run designed to make running both fun and productive, since these short all-out efforts will push your body to its limit and improve your speed in much the same way an interval workout can.

Warm-up: Either walk or run very slowly for the first 5 minutes of the workout.

Workout: 30-minute run in aerobic and tempo zone with several spontaneous bursts or sprints of various distances (but nothing that lasts more than 1 minute) thrown in during the middle portion. For example, pick a visual landmark ahead of you and run at a race pace or faster until you reach it—if you're running with a partner, race for it.

Cool-down: Walk for 5 minutes or run the last 5 minutes of your workout very slowly.

EVENING WORKOUTS

In my opinion, the evening workout is the one that requires the most self-discipline over the long haul, for one simple reason—hunger pains. Your evening workout window is somewhere between the time you get home and dinnertime, depending on what time you end your workday. Personally, I've always found it difficult to consistently get on the bike, hit the running trail, or dive into the pool after a tough day at work, facing the prospect of delaying my vittles for another hour or two. But on the occasions that I have mustered up the energy and conviction, I've found that an evening workout offers such benefits as these:

- It's a great time to leave the day's work or home pressure behind you and focus on some "me time."
- It reenergizes you for time later on with the family.
- Having dinner after a good workout encourages healthy eating habits and moderate food portions (and helps reduce the guilt factor from occasional cheating).
- It provides a springboard for a relaxing and enjoyable evening and a good night's sleep.

Preparation

The evening workout window is dependent on numerous variables, such as the time you get home, family responsibilities, and dinner plans. So it's all the more important to set aside this time and make a firm commitment to train before you sit down for your evening meal. That said, sometimes the world conspires to throw off your training, so have an alternative plan or an abbreviated workout in your back pocket, should you need it. Finding time to work out in the evening is important—whether before or after your dinner—so that you stay on track with your training.

Some hardy souls actually prefer to run later in the evening, such as after dinner. Nighttime runs can be invigorating. Make sure to take the appropriate safety precautions, such as wearing reflective clothing or a vest. Running in the evening can be dangerous in ways besides traffic—always stay away from secluded areas after dark. Again, you must find a time slot during the evening that balances your need to train with other demands on your time.

Consider starting your evening workouts immediately after you arrive home; have your workout clothes, gear, or gym bag ready to fly. It's best to avoid sitting down, watching television, or any sedentary activity that may lull you into skipping your workout. In fact, if it's convenient and feasible, go directly from your work to the health club or YMCA pool, running track, or bike trail before you go home—it then becomes the tail end of your commute. Just make sure you talk to your spouse or partner about changing your dinner plans so that you can fit in your evening workout—better yet, have them join you.

Getting in a bike workout at this time of day can be tough for two reasons: growing darkness and higher traffic on the roadways. Always use the appropriate safety precautions if you bike on the road.

Sample Evening Workouts

You have to be extremely flexible in planning your evening workouts. There are many variables to consider, so go easy on yourself if you have to notch it back (in intensity or distance) when other obligations or low energy reserves come into play.

▶ *EVENING SWIM WORKOUT (IRONMAN DISTANCE)*

Evening is a great time to swim, because it refreshes the body and mind late in the day and it's a perfect setup for a well-deserved meal.

Warm-up: 75 meters easy

Workout: Swim two 1900-meter segments with an easy to moderate effort; swim the first 1900 meters slightly more slowly than the second. Rest for 60 seconds between segments.

Cool-down: 75 meters easy

▶ *EVENING BIKE WORKOUT (OLYMPIC DISTANCE)*

Chances are you won't have much time in the evening to bike, since darkness may become a problem. Provided you can get in double-digit mileage or kilometers, this is a great workout that makes the best use of your time by pushing you into your aerobic zone for greater stamina.

Warm-up: 5 minutes spinning in an easy gear

Workout: 12 to 15 miles (19 to 24 kilometers) in aerobic and tempo zone

Cool-down: 5 minutes in an easy gear, then stretching your hamstrings and legs

▶ *EVENING RUN WORKOUT (SPRINT DISTANCE)*

This workout is relatively short and may be ideal for an after-meal run, since you do the first 10 minutes at an easy pace. The short interval of tempo running, however, also helps you work up a sweat and makes you feel as though you've accomplished some fitness gains (which you have).

Warm-up: Walk for 5 minutes or run the first 5 minutes of the workout very slowly.

Workout: 15-minute run, first 10 minutes easy with 5-minute tempo pace at the end (for a description of tempo pace running, see page 82 in the next chapter).

Cool-down: Walk for 5 minutes or run the last 5 minutes of your workout very slowly.

COMMUTING WORKOUTS

Substituting human-powered transportation for your typical work commute is one of the smartest and most innovative solutions for today's time-crunched, environmentally friendly triathlete. Although it's not a realistic option for everyone, cycling or running to work can be one of the most effective ways to consistently train during the work week with small to moderate time sacrifices (I have no doubt there are some triathletes out there who have managed to swim to work, but I'm speaking to the vast majority who don't work on a tug boat).

The savings on gas costs if you drive to work can even help pay for that new bike computer or new running shoes. You'll be protecting the ecosystem as well as sending a message that you care about the environment.

Sitting in bumper-to-bumper traffic while your hard-earned money seeps out your tailpipe can also start your day off on the wrong foot, leading to stress and a decidedly negative state of mind by the time you reach your destination. That's why more and more people, even nontriathletes seeking a better alternative, have turned to bicycle commuting. Whereas running is a more limited option (obviously much more dependent on distance to work), bicycle commuting is fast becoming a viable option. Many states sponsor trails or programs to encourage human-powered commutes.

Bicycling or running to work can help your triathlon training in many ways:

- Whether you tri-commute once, twice, or five times a week, these commuting distances contribute to your overall plan by adding distance that you might otherwise find much more difficult to fit into your busy schedule.

- Tri-commuting saves you money on transportation costs. In the United States, driving a car can cost 60 cents or more per mile, depending on the region, whereas bicycles, including repairs and maintenance, can average less than 10 cents per mile, potentially saving you thousands of dollars per year (Kifer 2002).

- You can reduce stress and arrive at your office or workplace physically energized and mentally refreshed.

- In some cases you may actually save time; depending on the route you choose and how fast you can ride, you may get to work faster on your bicycle.

Preparation

Commuting to work on your bicycle or by foot power takes some preparation in advance, and often requires trial and error to find the best route. Check local resources for bicycle trails and paths that may offer a more direct route than is possible by car, train, or bus. Always consider traffic on the route; it's always best to choose a route that may be more indirect but that offers the benefit of less traffic. Think of safety first when it comes to choosing the roadways for your commute. If you work normal hours, you'll probably find that your morning commute is less hectic than your afternoon commute (rush hour always seems to be more congested later in the day). Ride defensively and be careful out there.

You may also want to gradually make inroads into tri-commuting by limiting it to once or twice a week at first. If your commute is particularly demanding in terms of terrain or distance (or both), you'll want to limit these workouts to avoid overtraining.

If you're cycling, make sure your bicycle is in good working order and you have at least two spare tubes and everything you need to change a flat. If possible, time your commutes to avoid rush hour traffic. You'll need a durable, waterproof commuter backpack to carry a change of work clothes (unless you have access to a locker room or other similar facility at work or at a nearby health club).

When you're choosing a running route, pollution can be a problem. Car exhaust can actually be detrimental to your health if you pound the pavement near busy thoroughfares, so investigate possible paths away from traffic.

Sample Commuting Workouts

Your workout during a commute is obviously limited to the distance and course that you have chosen for getting to work. Deciding the pace and intensity that you'll execute during the commute will largely depend on your weekly goals, your current training stage, and how your workout fits with your other training. Ideas for commute training follow (with the exception of swimming). No race distances are given since the workout is dependent on the commuting distance.

▶ *COMMUTING BIKE WORKOUT*

Tailor the following workout as a recovery session or as training that helps build your fitness. Staying in the aerobic and tempo zone for as long as possible will improve both your endurance and stamina.

Warm-up: Spin in an easy gear for the first 10 minutes.

Workout: For a recovery workout, spin at 90 RPM or higher; for a harder workout, get into your aerobic and tempo zone and maintain your heart rate there for as much of the ride as possible (distance determined by commute).

Cool-down: Spin 5 minutes in an easy gear, then stretch your hamstrings and legs.

▶ *COMMUTING RUN WORKOUT*

Whether you live close enough to work to run all the way there or you jog from a train station to your job, you can adapt this workout to whatever fits best in your training schedule. Use it for recovery or a fun fartlek session that will improve your speed and technique.

Warm-up: Walk for 5 minutes or run the first 5 minutes of the workout very slowly.

Workout: Run at an easy pace the whole way (distance will depend on commute), or do some fartlek speed play and sprint for short distances several times during the middle of the run.

Cool-down: Walk for 5 minutes or run the last 5 minutes of your workout very slowly.

WEEKEND WORKOUTS

If you're like most people with a nine-to-five work schedule, you'll probably find that the biggest opportunity for crucial long rides and runs will be on the weekend. Yet with all the household chores, projects, errands, and so forth, you may find those crucial workouts fading into lost opportunities as you head back into the work week—unless, of course, you have a solid plan and you execute it.

In some ways, getting in your long weekend workouts takes more self-discipline than the shorter training you do during the week. Weekends give you more choices and freedom, and sometimes it's hard to say no to friends and family, let alone to your own temptation to skip that long run and watch the Sunday afternoon football game.

Remember that your ability to successfully juggle your other priorities in order to do critical long-distance training will have the biggest impact on your endurance and thus on your ability to achieve your triathlon goal. It's really as simple as that.

Weekend workouts are ideal for long rides and runs for many reasons:

- The potential to schedule longer blocks of training time on weekends allows you an opportunity to get in some significant distance.
- You're more likely to connect with training partners on weekends—absolutely indispensable for long bike rides and runs, when having companionship can help those miles or kilometers fly by in no time.
- More free time may allow you the opportunity to do cycling-running brick workouts, which will significantly improve your transition during races (provided you practice quick transitions from bike to run).
- Weekend trips or day trips to scenic running trails or better cycling roads can be much-needed occasional getaways.

Communication is vital if you need a significant slice of weekend time to complete your training. Family and friends need to know beforehand that training is a priority on the weekend and that—although you value your relationships with them—achieving your triathlon goal requires you to do what it takes, including spending significant time in the saddle and on the running path.

Training time is less of an issue for short-distance triathlons, since the training demands are fewer. You may well find that you need to supplement your weekday workouts with only slightly longer weekend workouts. In any case, once you've communicated your priorities to your significant others, the next key step is to assign a time slot to your training, much the way you would schedule an appointment with your doctor, vet, or hair salon.

Although the weekends give you flexibility, you may want to consider mornings as your best time of day to train on weekends. Morning workouts will free up the rest of your Saturdays and Sundays to enjoy time with your family and friends (and mow the lawn).

As with all your training, preparation and planning are the keys to weekend workouts. First, decide the best time of day for you to train on weekends and schedule a time slot. Second, make sure you communicate your commitment to triathlon training to affected friends and family. You can also explore opportunities to get your friends and family involved in your weekend training, such as getting your spouse to ride a bicycle alongside you on your long run, or attaching a tag-along buggy to your bicycle so that you can take your kids with you on a long ride. Third, be flexible and have a plan B in case circumstances don't allow you to make your workout appointment. Last, consider doing your long rides on Saturdays and long runs on Sundays, giving you the simulation of a triathlon over a two-day period with some time to recover in between. If you opt to do a difficult brick workout on Sundays, make sure you do an easy ride or pool workout on Saturday.

Literally any workout can be done on weekends. See the training plans in part III of this book for sample weekend workouts according to race distance.

GROUP WORKOUTS

Although not necessarily time based in nature, group workouts are worth mentioning as great alternatives to working out on your own or with the same training partners. Integrating group workouts into your schedule is a great time management strategy, because they occur at a fixed time. Because they are at fixed times and dates—usually on a weekly basis— Masters swim workouts, bike shop rides, or running club or store runs are great appointments on your training calendar that supplement your solo training.

Group workouts are also a smart way to consistently challenge yourself. You are quite likely to find yourself tested in the pool, on the roads, or on the trails, depending on your skill level, the discipline, and the group you're working out with.

Group workouts can be a genuine boost to your training:

- You can practically plan a sizable portion of your weekly training with group workouts (provided they are congruent with your goals).
- They require that you make time in your busy schedule and are usually planned for a time of day that is workable for most people.
- Training in groups may help to make a demanding session feel quick and effortless—you may even find time (and your heart rate) flying during that long ride or run.
- Humans are pack animals, and the social aspect of group training can make your triathlon experience more gratifying.

Although the advantages are real, a word of caution is warranted: Group training doesn't always meet your individual needs or match your current skill and fitness levels. Most Masters swim sessions, bike shop rides, and running groups are composed of athletes with a variety of skill and fitness levels. Even when there is a big gap between the slowest and the fastest, there is usually a structure that allows you to settle into a pack that is at your speed or training level.

For example, the weekly bike ride that starts every Wednesday evening at your local bicycle shop may include a few regulars who are category I or II riders (the highest rankings of cyclists that compete in United States Cycling Federation races) or top area triathletes. But there are probably more than a few middle-of-the-packers and a few recreational riders in the mix. Typically the group will split into subgroups according to level sometime during the ride, or a shop's policy may mandate that everyone stay together for safety reasons. In the latter scenario, a group ride leader may require everyone to wait for riders who fall behind at several intervals during the ride (which, admittedly, can be embarrassing if it's consistently you).

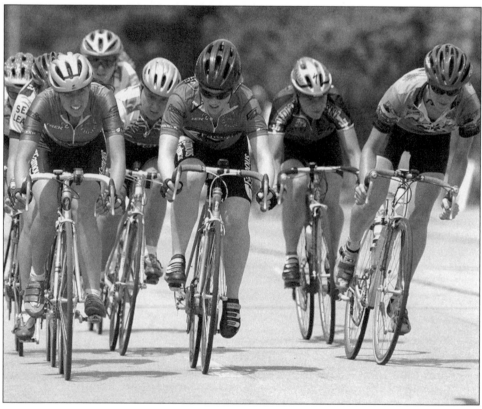

© Human Kinetics

A group workout can be a great alternative to working out on your own, provided it meets your individual training needs.

What's important is that you choose to work out with a group—in whichever discipline—that fits within the framework of your triathlon goal and your master plan. Pushing yourself too hard simply to save face and keep up with peers who are at a different level than you will only lead to burnout and potentially to injury.

Make sure to discuss your concerns and questions with the workout leader, especially if you're concerned you'll be pushing beyond your current level. For example, if it's a group ride out of a bike shop, will you know your way home if you get left behind? If a group run is at a distance too fast or too long for your current training, will you have the option to run with a slower group or cut it short? Most group workouts are designed to appeal to a wide range of ability, but discussing your concerns beforehand will help you be more at ease the first few times out.

To find swim group workouts in your area, call your local YMCA for Masters swim class information. For bike rides, visit a local, independently owned bike shop for information on weekly group rides—make sure they cater to triathletes at your level. Contact running specialty stores or area clubs for information on weekly group runs or track workouts.

One note—always arrive early to prepare for a group workout, especially for rides. Give yourself enough time to pump up your tires, lube your chain, and get your gear on (the last thing you want is a pack of angry cyclists waiting just for you).

CHAPTER **6**

Key Workouts

I'm sure you've had the experience of completing an especially good workout, one after which you felt confident you'd taken some large strides toward getting to where you need to be in order to achieve your triathlon race goal. Whether it was the distance, the intensity, or a potent combination of the two, these workouts seemed to outshine your other training.

It's not that every workout isn't important. The cumulative effect of hundreds of running and cycling miles or kilometers and thousands of pool meters is the sum total of your fitness. Even an easy 2-mile (3.2-kilometer) recovery run or a leisurely ride with your spouse has the benefit of consolidating the gains from your much harder workouts, helping to flush out lactic acid and keeping muscles loose. Unless you routinely train without a purpose, there are really no such things as garbage miles or meters.

Nevertheless, there are those few workouts that have a catalytic effect on your ability to swim, bike, and run faster or longer. Training timed properly and done at an intensity and distance that is ideal for meeting the demands of your race goal is what produces such results. It is training that is key.

In this chapter, we'll explore the key workout method and discuss how this approach can help you manage your triathlon time and increase your training efficiency.

KEY WORKOUTS EXPLAINED

Twenty-three-time Ironman champion Paula Newby-Fraser coined the phrase *key workouts* in her book *Peak Fitness for Women* (Newby-Fraser 1995). Like any triathlete or high-level fitness enthusiast, she was always strapped for time when trying to fit in all the training she felt was necessary for competing on the pro level. Whereas many of her counterparts engaged in hair-raising 500-mile bike weeks and killer 20-mile running workouts that would send even the most hard-core tri-geek hobbling to the freezer for an ice pack, she sought a better way.

Newby-Fraser noticed that there were a few triathletes who seemed to get it right consistently. They consistently raced well and, most important, never seemed to be tired or injured. She noticed that there was something common to all of their training regimens. The focus was not just on being out there and putting in the distances but also on a few particularly intense workouts that mirrored their individual performance goals.

After years of trial and error, Newby-Fraser found that she made the most of her time and training by simulating the conditions and intensity of competition as much as possible in a few select workouts. Some of these conditions included terrain, transitions, technical skills, and even eating and hydrating.

Based on dozen of interviews with fellow pros and her own personal findings, Newby-Fraser developed the key workout method that featured one crucial workout per week in each of the three disciplines, an approach that allowed for optimal performance and exercise recovery. Although there were some exceptions, any greater frequency per week of these demanding workouts appeared to tax the body beyond an ability to recover; any less yielded little performance improvement.

If you adopt the key workout approach to training, there will be three or four sessions that you should consider the core of your training schedule each week, usually one in each discipline. This handful of sessions will be the best measure of your fitness and the acid test for speed, endurance, and strength. After a key workout, you should be able to accurately judge where you are on your own performance scale. Some judge their performance by miles or meters covered, but total distance alone may camouflage weaknesses, such as lack of speed, endurance, or strength. Key workouts are performed at an intensity or a distance (or both) that—if successfully executed—gives you an accurate measuring stick of your current fitness.

Key workouts depend heavily on consistently planning your training in advance and adjusting it weekly. Although this is true for all training, key workouts are at a significant level of intensity or distance, making it crucial to plan both them and the intervening workouts to avoid overtraining. Sitting down at the end of a week to plan the next seven days is critical to the success of these workouts, because these three or four workouts become your performance scale and your true-north compass for the following week.

As with all your training, the make-up of your key workouts depends largely on what stage of your overall training plan you're in. For example, the swimming, cycling, and running you do during base training—when you are focusing on building a foundation of endurance and stamina—is exclusively distance work with low intensity and little or no intervals. Planning your workouts week to week within the larger framework of your seasonal training calendar ensures that your key workouts are right in line with your goal.

Next we'll tackle the key workout method for each of the three disciplines, including descriptions of some sample workouts that you can easily integrate into your own training plan. Swimming adds drills as a chief component of key workouts, because it is a sport that relies mainly on solid technique for improvement.

KEY SWIMMING WORKOUTS

Most triathletes come from an endurance sport background; the majority have the most experience in running. Like many triathletes, I graduated from spending a few years finishing about a dozen marathons to dipping my toe into multisports. I sought a new challenge and a better way to stay physically fit and injury free through cross-training. Swimming was the one discipline that presented the biggest test for me, because it was not just about being able to endure. It was about technique. In fact, the mistakes many triathletes make when planning their swim training can be attributed to their established view of how to get better at cycling and running—the more and longer you go, the better. But because of the highly technical nature of swimming, which involves an arm stroke, leg kick, head turn, horizontal body positioning, breathing pattern, hip turn, and a number of other movements, just doing it longer doesn't guarantee results.

As with a tennis backhand that consistently loses you points or a golf stroke that finds you flailing in the brush, practicing swimming with bad technique only guarantees that you'll learn to swim badly longer. Worse, consistently practicing poor swimming technique creates a deeper muscle memory groove that will become ingrained in your body.

The importance of technique is why swimming key workouts should consistently focus on a combination of technique drills and interval training. Intervals are multiple, short, moderate- to high-intensity bursts of effort over a measured distance, with a specified recovery time between each interval or repeat. Intervals are expressly designed to condition your body on several different levels to swimming (or cycling or running, as discussed further in the next chapter) at a faster pace with improved technique and increasing endurance. For less experienced swimmers, drills that help develop good technique should make up a portion of your workout during the earlier training stages, such as base training. Advanced swimmers with solid skills need to work primarily on interval training, but they also benefit from the occasional drill set to help keep their technique crisp and efficient.

Mathew Luebbers, head coach for the Marine Corps Semper Fit Aquatics Okinawa Dolphins swim team in Japan, recommends a combination of specific drills and key workouts for improving swimming technique. His program for a triathlete focuses on key swim workouts that involve race simulation, swimming skill proficiency, sustainable swimming speed, and time to recover after a swim. "Work on technique, work on going faster, work on holding good technique while going faster, but don't work on only one of these elements. They are all important," says Coach Mat.

An improvement in skill level can show up in at least two ways. You can swim a distance in a lower number of strokes in the same time, or you can swim a distance in the same number of strokes in a lower time. Both are good.

Swimming Technique Drills

If swimming is your weakest link, it is probably to a great degree because of lack of good technique in the pool. The good news is that technique is an issue that you can resolve. The bad news—depending on how long you've been swimming with poor strokes or balance—is that it can take a lot of work over an extended period of time to undo bad habits and replace them with good ones.

The trick is to make swim drills a standard part of your workouts. You can even use drill sets as a warm-up and cool-down for your interval workouts or for long swims. This powerful combination makes for more efficient, effective training. The key is that you tackle individual drills on a regular basis until you master them and move on to another. Don't be discouraged—swimming is a highly technical activity. It takes persistence, time, and patience before all that work translates into seconds and then minutes off your swim times.

The following drills provided by Coach Mat will help you improve your swimming technique, giving you greater confidence and comfort in open water. Proficient swimmers often say that the swim leg of a triathlon is too short, whereas nonswimmers say the opposite. According to Coach Mat, this disparity has a lot to do with the level of technical proficiency of the swimmer, not necessarily with the swimmer's fitness.

Swimming drills are specific movements, done repetitively, to get your technique in the groove. They can help you get faster and more efficient. Here are just a few of my favorites.

▶ CATCH-UPS

This drill helps isolate one arm to practice a long stroke and a long body position. Swim as in regular freestyle, except that one arm is stationary, always extending forward and pointing toward the destination (front arm), while the other arm performs the stroke (working arm). When the working arm moves forward and catches up with the stationary arm, they change places.

Variations:

- **3/4 catch-up:** Just like full catch-up, except the stationary (front) arm begins to work or move before the other arm fully catches up. It begins to move after the working arm is about three-quarters of the way through a full arm motion.

- **Catch-up with a board:** Just like regular catch-up, only your front hand is holding a kickboard; as the arms trade places, they hand off the board to each other. The board lets you focus on one arm at a time, helping you pinpoint any flaws in your technique as you switch from your dominant hand to your nondominant side.

▶ *FINGERTIP DRAG*

This drill helps to promote a high-elbow recovery and to make you aware of your hand position during recovery. Swim regular freestyle, except that your fingertips never leave the water as your arm moves forward during the stroke recovery. You drag your fingers forward through the water, slightly off to the side of your body, focusing on good body roll and keeping your elbows pointed up. Vary how much of your hand stays in the water: fingertips, hand, wrist, even your whole forearm.

▶ *FIST*

This drill develops your feel for the water by getting you in tune with how cupping your hand can affect how fast you propel yourself forward. Swim your regular freestyle stroke, but hold one or both of your hands in a fist instead of using your normal cupped hand. Vary the pattern and the number of strokes for which you are fisted. When you unclench your hand, you should notice a difference in pressure on your hand; use this feeling to fine-tune how you cup the water as you propel yourself forward while you move through your pull pattern. When your fist is clenched, you should also try to press on the water with the inside (palm side) of your forearm—think of the lower arm, from elbow to wrist, as an extension of your hand. And don't forget to watch body roll.

▶ *ONE-ARM*

This drill helps you to focus on one arm at a time. Swim regular freestyle, except that only one arm is moving. The other arm is stationary, either forward (front hand) or backward against your side (back hand). The moving hand takes a series of strokes; each arm performs a set number of pulls before it switches roles with the other. Practice this drill with the stationary arm in both positions. When your stationary arm is at your side, breathe toward that side (away from the moving arm). When your stationary arm is forward, breathe away from it (toward the arm doing the work). Again, time the breathing so that as your body rolls, your head rolls with it for a breath, and then your head should return to its forward alignment.

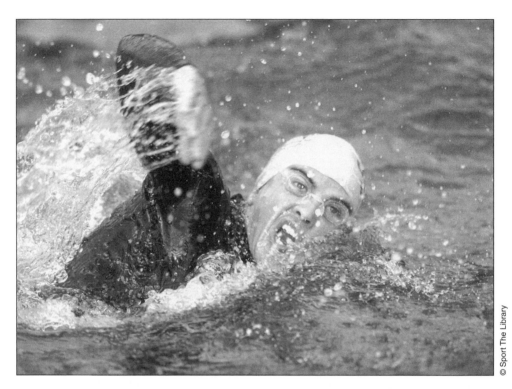

© Sport The Library

Key swimming workouts that combine technique drills and interval training will make you a fierce competitor in the water.

Sample Key Swimming Workouts

This section features sample key swim workouts provided by Coach Mat that fall into seven different categories. Each category emphasizes a different important aspect of swimming critical to triathlon success. The categories are detailed as follows with specific examples for various distances (see chapters 8 to 11 for swim workouts for all the major triathlon distances).

▶ *BRAINWORK*

This workout takes plenty of concentration because you aim to maintain a steady pace while achieving a high level of technical proficiency. Although it sounds easy, maintaining the same pace throughout the distance can be mentally and technically challenging, but it is well worth the benefits on race day. Target speed is race pace or slower, but always the same speed through the entire swim.

Frequency: Every 2 to 3 weeks

Sample workout (sprint distance): 750-meter swim with a steady, sustainable, nonstop effort. Your total time should go down as you get fitter; you might also find that your time stays the same but you feel stronger at the end of the swim, an indicator of increased technical proficiency. Over time, add 100 to 300 meters to these swims until you cover the full distance that you'll be racing.

▶ *RACE SIMULATION*

Every race has cycles of intensity within each discipline, and swimming is no different. This workout is designed to simulate a rapid (sometimes high-intensity) swim start, a moderate and steady tempo during the middle meters, and a slightly higher pace toward the end when you would normally be eager to reach the shore. It's subtle, but these kinds of simulations help prepare you for the real thing. Target speed is race pace.

Frequency: Every 4 to 6 weeks

Sample workout (Olympic distance): 1500-meter swim with varied efforts to simulate the early, middle, and late portions of the race. Swim the first 50 strokes at a moderate to high level, the middle portion at a moderate, sustainable level, and the closing section at a moderate to moderately higher level (not as fast as the first 50 strokes). At the end of this swim, check your heart rate; check it again at 30, 60, and 90 seconds. As you get fitter, your heart rate should go down faster or your total swim time will get faster.

▶ *TECHNIQUE GOLF*

This workout helps you reduce your stroke count by likening it to the rules of golf, making it a fun exercise to improve your swimming. Vary speeds from slower, to faster than race pace, to experiment with stroke rate, stroke distances, and so forth. As experience is gained, you'll either move to a narrower stroke range and toward race pace or you'll swim from slightly slower early in the set to race pace or faster later in the set.

Frequency: Every week

Sample workout (half-Ironman distance): Swim 10 × 25 meters (or 50 meters), resting 15 to 30 seconds between lengths and counting strokes for each length. Add stroke count and time in seconds. Aim to decrease total for each 25 (or 50) meters within a workout and over the weeks.

▶ *SUSTAINABLE PACE*

These workouts are designed to bring your fitness level close to what you'll need to finish your swim leg feeling strong. Target speed is to average race pace, with the variation between segments narrowing with experience.

Frequency: Every 1 to 2 weeks

Sample workout (Ironman distance): Divide the race distance into two parts (2 × 1900 meters). Swim the first segment at an easy to moderate effort that results in a time slower than segment two. Rest for 60 seconds, checking every 20 seconds to see whether you are recovering. If your heart rate is not going down, continue resting and checking every 20 seconds until it starts to go down, then wait an additional 20 seconds before starting the second part. As you gain fitness, attempt to swim each segment at an equal pace and then attempt to decrease the rest between segments. Don't try to accomplish both goals at the same time. Focus on increasing the pace for segment one first.

▶ HOLD A PACE

This demanding workout will help you make solid gains in your fitness level while you continue to seek a high level of technical proficiency. Target speed is the fastest possible speed you can sustain for all repeats.

Frequency: Every 2 to 4 weeks

Sample workout (Olympic distance): 10 × 50 meters with 10 seconds rest between intervals, at the fastest possible even pace. Swim all intervals at the same speed, with the goal of feeling as though you might be able to do one or two more once you finish the set, but no more. At the end of this swim, check your heart rate; check it again at 30, 60, and 90 seconds. As you get fitter, your heart rate should go down faster or your total swim time should get faster.

▶ COUNTDOWN

By starting with the longest interval distance at a slower pace to the shortest interval at the fastest pace, you'll gain a feel for how critical good technique can be in improving your speed. The target is to average race pace, starting below race pace and ending faster than race pace so that the variance narrows with experience.

Frequency: Every 4 to 6 weeks

Sample workout (half-Ironman distance): Swim 1900 meters as a 550, 450, 350, 250, 150, 100, 50; rest 10 to 20 seconds between each segment. Aim to go faster as the segments get shorter. Over time, aim to decrease total swim time.

▶ HARD-EASY-HARD

These workouts build in a recovery interval between hard efforts to help you improve your stamina during a race. Target speed is as fast as you can go for four sets in a row. Speed may decrease 5 to 10 seconds from first to fourth set and from fifth to eighth set, but if the slowdown is greater, then your speed is too great.

Frequency: Every 1 to 2 weeks

Sample workout (sprint or Olympic distance): Swim 4 × 50 meters at a fast, sustainable speed; 2 × 50 meters very easy focusing on technique; and 4 × 50 meters at a fast, sustainable speed, all on 30 to 60 seconds rest between intervals. At the end of this set, check your heart rate; check it again at 30, 60, and 90 seconds. As you get fitter, your fast times should get faster, and your heart rate should recover faster.

KEY CYCLING WORKOUTS

Among amateur triathletes, the cycling portion of a race is often underestimated. It is hands down the most critical leg of a race, and not just because it is typically the longest. A weakness on the bike can drastically bump you down in the standings very quickly. But what many triathletes don't consider is how harmful a lack of cycling fitness or a strategic error (such as riding in a gear that's too hard) can be to your running success.

In my early days of competing in triathlons, my lifelong friend and relay teammate, Guillermo, would occasionally compete head-to-head with me in a 10K, half-marathon, or marathon. Invariably I would get beat, especially the longer the running distance. However, I almost always had the better of him during a triathlon. Our swimming ability was equal because we had learned to swim properly together as adults, specifically to compete in triathlons, and we both started from ground zero. But Guillermo always gravitated toward running whereas I spent the greater portion of my training on the bike.

You might think my lead off the bike would evaporate on the run. However, Guillermo's running strength would inevitably be negated by his dead, tired legs. Whereas under marathon circumstances I would be chased down within miles, in triathlons my running on fresher, fitter legs off the bike allowed me to hold my own and minimize any gains Guillermo might make on me.

One of my favorite race photos shows me yards from the finish line of the Chicago Triathlon years ago. Instead of looking forward toward the finish, the photo shows me looking back, straining to see whether Guillermo was right on my heels. My longtime friend was miles behind me, having underestimated the importance of proper cycling training.

Whether you consider yourself a hammer king or count yourself among the cursed on a bike leg, focusing on some key workouts can not only help you increase the pace you can maintain throughout a race, it can also set you up nicely with some relatively fresh legs for a really great run. Cycling offers the triathlete a variety of options when it comes to training. You can use variables such as the degree of difficulty of a course, pace, and distance to help you meet your individual needs. There are also some great training aids, such as rollers, that can really help you improve your technique for more efficient power output on the bike.

Steven Truesdale, cycling coach at Colorado Performance Coaching, has identified certain key workouts that consistently provide significant performance benefits to the triathletes he coaches. Here Coach S.T. presents a few examples of key cycling workouts in various distances.

These demanding workouts, organized by distance, will improve not only your fitness but also your pedaling technique. Although not as critical as in swimming, cycling technique does play a vital role during a triathlon because of the importance of energy conservation. Poor pedaling technique can make you expend more energy and, more important, can lead to knee and back injuries. Here you'll find a good combination of technique-based workouts and, of course, some challenging riding.

Note: Some of the following workouts refer to RPM (revolutions per minute), which will require a cycling computer with cadence feature.

Sprint or Olympic Distance

For triathletes training for Olympic- or sprint-distance races there are three important bike workouts that I consider key, for any time during the base or peak training periods. Two of the three workouts are relatively easy and focus on technique, so you can consider each key and still do them weekly.

▶ *HEART RATE WORKOUT (SPRINT OR OLYMPIC DISTANCE)*

During sprint-distance triathlons, the bike leg is short and can be done at very high intensity, if a racer is well prepared. This is a great short, intense workout designed to increase your anaerobic endurance and recovery. It can be done on the road or on a trainer.

Warm-up: Cycle easy for up to 15 minutes at approximately 90 RPM, gradually raising your heart rate from your recovery and endurance zone to your aerobic and tempo zone.

Workout: Do 4 to 6 intervals at a very high intensity, building to the upper end of your anaerobic threshold zone. The first interval should be 2 minutes. Increase each successive interval by 30 seconds to a maximum of 4 minutes. Rest up to 1 minute between intervals, or enough to allow a heart rate recovery back down into your aerobic and tempo zone.

Cool-down: Ride 10 to 15 minutes, doing easy recovery spinning in your recovery and endurance zone.

▶ *PEDALING EFFICIENCY WORKOUT*

For new triathletes preparing for a sprint-distance race, pedaling efficiency is often an area that needs attention. Proper pedaling technique and increased efficiency allow the racer to maximize her power and speed. This workout is designed to improve pedaling efficiency and smoothness, a key cycling skill for all levels. It can be done on a trainer at home or on a long flat section of road.

Warm-up: Pedal slow and easy for 10 to 15 minutes at a comfortable RPM of about 80.

Workout: Choose a low to moderate gear that allows high-RPM pedaling. Over the course of 30 seconds, slowly increase RPM from 80 to as high as you can go without bouncing up out of the saddle. Hold this high RPM for 5 to 10 seconds, and then rest for a minute. Repeat this high-RPM drill 5 to 10 times. During the drill, try to maintain a focus on a smooth and efficient pedaling style—stay seated and keep your upper body from moving around too much. As you get more comfortable with high-RPM pedaling, try to maintain the high RPM level as long as you can.

Cool-down: Finish with a very easy 10-minute cool-down period.

▶ ROLLER WORKOUT

This workout is a skill drill appropriate for all riders but is especially important for new riders unfamiliar with technique. By means of the sink-or-swim circumstance that riding on rollers can provide, this workout increases competencies such as pedaling technique, smoothness, and overall cycling confidence.

In case you're unfamiliar with rollers, they are a type of trainer in which the bike is placed on a set of small-diameter, 16-inch-wide drums that roll on bearings. The drums are attached to a frame. The front wheel of the bike spins at the same rate as the back wheel, because the front drum is attached by a rubber band looped through one of the back rollers. The rider maintains an upright position because of the gyroscopic action of the wheels—the same as riding on the road. A basic set of rollers are available online for as little as $125.

Many find riding rollers to be difficult at first, so to start with, place the rollers inside a door frame so that you can have one hand on the door frame while riding and steadying the bike. Mount the bike with one brake on to keep the wheels from rolling. Once seated, with one hand on the door frame and one hand on the brakes, slowly pedal to rotate the wheels. Keep riding smoothly and steadily. Once you master them, riding rollers will become second nature and result in smoother and more efficient pedaling on the road.

Warm-up and initial workout: Once you are able to mount the bike and ride for a short period without wallowing left and right across the front drum, take your hand off the door frame and put it on the bars. Keep your eyes forward, watch your steering, and keep the pedaling smooth. You will soon master the technique, so keep trying. Work until you can do 10 minutes straight on the rollers. This may be all you can do at first and may be your entire workout, so don't be discouraged—it is an acquired skill that takes patience and time.

Subsequent workouts: When you can master 10 minutes of riding on rollers, consider moving them to the center of a room and placing a chair next to them to assist you in mounting the bike. Then ride while trying to move your hands around on the bars. Try reaching down for a water bottle. Try shifting up and down gears and finding an RPM that you are comfortable with. Try some pedaling cadence changes—up and down—70 to 90 RPM. Work at it until you can ride a set of rollers smoothly for 30 minutes, while changing gears, shifting weight, and drinking from a bottle with one hand. After a couple of weeks you will be able to ride smoothly and efficiently. Because the drums are only so wide, you are forced to stay smooth and calm and efficient in order to stay on the rollers. Riding rollers increases your pedaling smoothness, and thus makes you a faster, more efficient cyclist.

Cool-down: Ride the rollers at a smooth, easy pace for 5 to 10 minutes.

Olympic or Half-Ironman Distance

For triathletes training for Olympic to half-Ironman races there are two important bike workouts that are key during an 8- to 12-week prerace buildup period. These can be done every week, one time each, as two key bike workouts.

▶ SPEED WORKOUT

This is a great midweek speed workout designed to build good pedaling cadence while working on power. You can do it on a trainer at home or sneak out of the office for a lunchtime ride.

Warm-up: Ride about 15 minutes in the saddle at approximately 90 RPM, gradually building from your recovery and endurance zone to your aerobic and tempo zone.

Workout: Ride 60 minutes, shorter for a lunch ride. Do 5 to 10 sprints of 30 seconds each. For each sprint, start off in a higher gear with a lower RPM of about 70 and power your way to a fast RPM sprint. Don't worry about your heart rate. As a matter of fact, don't even look at your heart rate monitor—it might scare you. Recover well in between sprints.

Cool-down: Do a 10- to 15-minute easy recovery spin.

▶ ENDURANCE RIDE

This workout is the long endurance ride for the week. It is designed to build aerobic and muscular endurance. Find a 2- to 3-hour bike ride that simulates your race route to some degree.

Warm-up: Ride at a slow, easy pace for 20 to 30 minutes at approximately 90 RPM.

Workout: Maintain a steady 90 to 120 minutes in your aerobic and tempo zone. Stay in the aero position for as much of this period as you can, and get out of the saddle only for short periods of time on hills. Be careful about spending much time at the upper range of your target zone, and completely avoid going anaerobic.

Cool-down: Finish with a very easy 15- to 20-minute cool-down period in your recovery and endurance zone.

Ironman Distance

For triathletes training for Ironman-distance races there are two bike workouts that are key during the 10- to 12-week buildup period before the prerace taper—one is a hill workout, the other a race simulation brick. The hill workout is included in this section. The race simulation brick can be found in the next chapter on page 97. These workouts can be done on alternating Saturdays, depending on your schedule, for a minimum of five times each during your peak training phase and before tapering off your training before race day.

▶ *HILL WORKOUT*

The hill workout is a long bike workout that combines functions that are designed to build aerobic and muscular endurance as well as power. Map out a hilly course for this ride, preferably one where you won't start any significant climbing until about 60 to 90 minutes into the ride. Plan on spending 4 hours or more on this workout, depending on your individual fitness, your schedule, and how long it is until your race. Although this is a large chunk of time, it's typical for an Ironman-distance workout. It's also still efficient in that the course and intensity of the middle miles provide a great way to build your fitness and leg strength. The closer you get to your target Ironman-distance race, the longer this workout should be. To add time to this ride, repeat stages 2 and 3 of the workout. This is a great group training ride—invite your race buddies along.

Warm-up: Cycle at a slow, easy pace for an hour at approximately 90 RPM. Keep your intensity low and begin to hydrate and eat (even if you're not feeling thirsty or hungry).

Workout stage 1: Increase the intensity a bit, and maintain a steady 45 to 60 minutes in the upper range of your recovery and endurance zone and into the bottom range of your aerobic and tempo zone, putting you at about 70 to 80 percent of your maximum heart rate. At the end of this time you should be at the bottom of a long hill.

Workout stage 2: Divide the climb into three sections, each one-third of an hour-long climb, or 3 × 20 minutes. In the first climbing set (20 minutes), spin up the climb in a low gear and enter your aerobic and tempo zone. Then recover and start the second climb, doing it at a moderate effort. Pick a big gear that allows a relatively low yet still comfortable RPM, such as 65 to 70. Climb 3 × 6 minutes hard in the saddle, and really push it into your anaerobic threshold zone. Do the third 20 minutes of climbing the same as the first 20 minutes, back into the aerobic and tempo zone. Stay hydrated and continue eating.

Workout stage 3: Head for home, doing the fourth hour of this ride at your race pace. Avoid any high intensity during this portion. Stay steady, ride strong, and keep the RPM high.

Cool-down: Do 30 minutes of very easy riding.

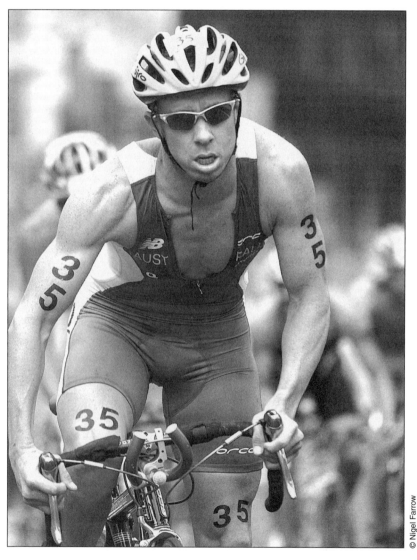

© Nigel Farrow

The cycling portion of a race is the most critical, and it can make or break your success in the running leg.

KEY RUNNING WORKOUTS

If you've ever read about, invested in, or talked to an expert about the stock market, chances are there's one phrase you've heard quite often: Diversify, diversify, diversify. A healthy stock portfolio that minimizes risk and maximizes returns is usually one that contains a balanced mix of investments.

Similarly, if you want to realize some fitness dividends and good race time returns, you've got to diversify your triathlon training and make sure your key workouts result in a balanced approach to running fitness. Just as a portfolio includes a mix of conservative, moderate, and aggressive investments, your run training should comprise a combination of workouts that build endurance, stamina, speed, and your ability to recover.

If running is an area of your triathlon training that you need to focus on and improve, the good news is that there are plenty of ways you can boost your speed. It may be challenging to tackle some workouts that force you to leave your comfort zone and push yourself to an intensity that you may not be used to. Running workouts, like the intervals and even tempo runs detailed in this section, are not easy, but they will, over time, increase your ability to push yourself to faster and faster times.

Pay special attention to your technique, especially during high-intensity or long runs. When you are fatigued, it's easy to lose your proper form. Maintaining good form under duress is a mental skill that you can carry over into any triathlon discipline, and it is a worthy skill to master. If you catch yourself slumping forward too much when you run, striking the pavement awkwardly, or running downhill looking like you're out of control, practice snapping back into form. Visualize yourself running as though you are running mile one. With continued diligence, you'll recognize the times when you slip into bad form and be able to get your running back on track.

There is no greater feeling during a race than gliding through the last few miles of a triathlon course and running strongly to the finish. The following workouts are designed to help you do just that. Here you'll find the guidelines you need to ensure that you plan each type of running key workout, in terms of frequency and distance, for your best running returns. For example, use the percentage of weekly distance figures to determine the number of miles or meters you should be running each specific type of workout. Once you've done that, you can determine how many workouts per week of each type to do and schedule them appropriately in your training calendar.

▶ *LONG SLOW DISTANCE RUNNING (LSD)*

Pace: Conservative—you should have enough breath to be able to hold a conversation relatively easily.

Percentage of weekly distance: 25 to 40 percent

Return: Endurance

If you do them once a week, you can accomplish long steady runs at an easy, comfortable intensity or at a pace you consider comfortably hard (is that an oxymoron?) Run at a pace that you can maintain for an hour or two without struggling to breathe. You've probably heard of the talk test, and your ability to sustain a conversation is actually a pretty good indicator of the correct long slow distance pace.

You should be working at what you perceive to be 60 to 70 percent of your maximum effort. This intensity, coupled with long continuous effort, is ideal for developing the cardiovascular system, improving the blood flow in active muscles, and increasing overall fitness and strength.

▶ *TEMPO RUNNING*

Pace: Moderate

Percentage of weekly distance: 20 to 30 percent

Return: Stamina

Tempo running is running at a fairly fast pace that you can maintain for 20 to 30 minutes, 15 to 20 seconds slower than your fastest 10K pace. The purpose of tempo runs is to take your body to the edge of what's called your lactate threshold, the point beyond which blood lactic acid begins accumulating at a more rapid rate.

You may have experienced going beyond your lactate threshold when climbing a hill, or when getting on a stair stepper and feeling a burn in your thighs. Tempo runs are designed to push your threshold further and further away so that eventually your body is able to tolerate a faster pace without lactic acid buildup.

Tempo runs stress your body to a certain point—not less, not more. Keep in mind that hills, uneven footing, and strong winds can affect intensity, so try to run them on a flat, even course. Depending on your level of fitness, do either one or two of these workouts per week.

▶ *INTERVAL OR SPEED WORK TRAINING*

Pace: Aggressive

Percentage of weekly distance: 10 to 20 percent

Return: Speed

Interval runs are repeated short bursts of speed over a measured distance (usually on a track), with recovery periods of either walking or relaxed jogging in between. Whether you walk or jog doesn't matter much. What's more important is that you give yourself sufficient time to recover between intervals. A 1:1 interval-recovery ratio is a good rule of thumb.

The purpose of interval running is to increase your maximum oxygen uptake, and the faster running teaches your body to be more biomechanically efficient. One interval workout a week is plenty, and you should schedule it with easy days before and after for recovery.

Many types of interval workouts are possible, so your workout should reflect your individual fitness level. If in doubt, err on the side of caution and start slowly with two or three quarter-mile intervals, running at your fastest 5K pace, with one recovery lap between each hard effort. You can add one interval per week and get creative with your workout later on, running so-called pyramids or perhaps a mile relay with a group of runners. Interval work is such an important part of training that the next chapter will address this topic in greater detail.

Once you reach a good fitness level you can add another day of speed work, but try to make it away from the track. A good alternative is a tempo run with some spontaneous, high-intensity bursts, described in the previous chapter as fartlek or speed play.

▶ *RECOVERY RUNS, CROSS-TRAINING, OR A DAY OFF*

Pace: Conservative

Percentage of weekly distance: 10 to 20 percent

Return: Recovery

After a particularly hard workout for you, whether it be any of the types of sessions listed previously or others, consider going for a short- or medium-distance run at a relaxed, easy pace. Better yet, an easy day of cycling or a few laps in the pool can do wonders to rejuvenate your beat-up body. If you are feeling particularly poor or sluggish, it is best to take the day off.

CHAPTER 7

80/20 Workouts

Triathlon training is like anything else in life—the greater your ability to focus on what's most important, the greater your success. Your ability to execute the most critical workouts that yield the most significant benefits has the most direct and dramatic impact on your fitness, your technique, and ultimately your race results. These workouts may represent only 20 percent or so of your total regimen, but they are probably responsible for 80 percent of your fitness, stamina, power, and technical skills.

Why are 80/20 workouts so effective? Because in most cases you do them at a high level of intensity, duration, or both, which helps you achieve significant gains in your overall fitness and ability to perform at your best during a triathlon. The 80/20 workouts that target weaknesses or technical skills in your sport are effective because they challenge you to shore up the flaws in your execution or discipline that cause you the greatest amount of harm during a triathlon.

Whereas the previous chapter detailed a variety of key workouts to plan weekly in each discipline, this chapter puts a smaller handful of proven workouts under the magnifying glass for closer scrutiny. Any of these workouts can be considered key workouts (for example, I discussed intervals in the previous chapter but do so here in further detail). However, some of these 80/20 workouts may be too rigorous to complete every week. Some are fashioned around your race distance and specific challenges of the course, whereas others are determined by your weakest discipline or lack of good technique. They are all essential weapons in your training arsenal, and you should execute them at strategic times during your schedule.

Planning 80/20 workouts strategically means making sure that you include the ones that help you improve your technique and shore up weakness early in your training season, preferably as you build your foundation during base training. It also means planning slots in your training season for bricks and some of the other challenging workouts you'll learn about here that will help you peak for race day but also give you enough time to recover.

INTERVALS

Intervals (also known as repeats) are short bursts of speed repeated over a measured distance with recovery periods between each interval. As I discussed in the previous chapter, intervals are a key component of training for swimming and running. In this chapter, we'll further explore 80/20 running workouts and also learn how to apply interval training to cycling.

Elite runner and author Jeff Galloway once wrote, "Intervals are based on a simple principle: The only way to run faster is to run faster" (Galloway 1984). Although that premise is true, there are some specific guidelines to interval training that can help you prevent injury and get the most out of your hard work.

• **Base training first.** Never begin any kind of speed work without a year's solid base of consistent distance running. Intervals are demanding and can be very rough on your body, so it's important that you've developed the muscle strength and joint integrity to support the effort.

• **Set a baseline with a time trial.** It's a good idea to start off your interval training with a performance benchmark that tells you where you are now so that you can measure your speed improvements down the road. To set a baseline with a time trial, warm up at a slow pace for 2 miles (3.2 kilometers) on a running track that's at least a quarter-mile (0.4 kilometer) long so that you don't have the constant turning. Perform a 1-mile (1.6-kilometer) time trial at a hard pace you can sustain throughout the entire distance. Time yourself with a stopwatch (or have somebody time you). Cool down for another 2 miles (3.2 kilometers) of easy jogging. Make sure you record your trial time (not including warm-up or recovery distance) in your training log. Once every other month, repeat your 1-mile time trials, and you should see some steady, measurable improvements.

• **Train for your distance.** The interval workout for an Ironman-distance triathlon is much different than that for a sprint distance. For example, if you're training for an Ironman-distance triathlon, you should be running half-mile (0.8-kilometer) intervals, 1-mile (1.6-kilometer) intervals, or a combination of both. This regimen builds your stamina and improves form for longer distances. For Olympic- or sprint-distance races, your workout should consist of a combination of half-mile (0.8-kilometer) and quarter-mile (0.4-kilometer) repeats.

• **Sandwich intervals with easy workouts.** Speed work is very demanding, so you need to be relatively fresh going into one and give yourself a day or two of easy work afterward.

• **Base your speed on your best running race times.** Most intervals come in three distances: quarter-, half-, or 1-mile (0.4-, 0.8-, or 1.6-kilometer) intervals. How fast should you run them? You should feel as though you're running close to your redline of effort, but err on the side of caution. If you feel as if you're blowing a gasket, ease off. For a quarter-mile interval, run 5 to 7 seconds faster than your 5K to 10K race pace. For a half-mile interval, you should run at 5K pace to 5 seconds faster. For a mile interval, you should run at 5K to 10K pace.

• **Increase gradually.** The first time on a track (once you've done a proper warm-up and a performance benchmark time trial as previously described) you'll want to start with only one or two repeats. It may even seem like an easy or short workout at first, but err on the side of caution. Gradually increase the number of intervals according to your race distance and goal.

• **Watch your form.** The tendency for some triathletes is to lose proper running form after a long and arduous bike leg. Track workouts are an ideal time to focus on your form and make an effort to keep your body under control during sustained, high-intensity efforts. Similar to proper technique in the pool, good running form helps you become more efficient and avoid injury with good biomechanics. If you feel yourself running awkwardly or find your feet striking the track improperly during the latter half of an interval workout, consciously bring your body back to running smoothly and effortlessly.

• **Aim for consistent interval times.** Done properly, interval workouts help your body to adapt to the prolonged hard effort of the running leg of a triathlon. By "properly" I mean a consistent pace on all the intervals. If there is more than a 5-second difference between interval times, you're probably going out too fast for the first few. You need to hone your internal pace clock, which is in itself a valuable skill to have during any running event.

▶ SAMPLE RUNNING INTERVAL WORKOUT— OLYMPIC DISTANCE

Come to the track prepared for a hard workout and equipped with plenty of fluids so that you can hydrate properly. You should have taken an easy day or two off so that you feel fresh and ready to run hard.

Warm-up: Run 1 to 2 miles (1.6 to 3.2 kilometers) around the track at an easy, conversational pace.

Workout stage 1: Run two quarter-mile (0.4-kilometer) intervals at 5 to 7 seconds faster than your average 10K race pace—make sure to fully recover between intervals.

Workout stage 2: Run one half-mile (0.8-kilometer) interval at your average 5K race pace, and then recover.

Workout stage 3: Run one or two (depending on fitness) quarter-mile intervals at 5 to 7 seconds faster than your average 10K race pace—recover between intervals.

Cool-down: Run 1 mile around the track, and walk for half a mile.

Modification: If you're new to track intervals, a good modification would be to simply skip stage 2 (the half-mile interval).

Although athletes most often associate intervals with running on a track, you can employ this type of speedwork just as easily on the bicycle, with great success. Professional cyclists have known for decades that a track isn't always necessary for interval work.

▶ SAMPLE CYCLING INTERVAL TRAINING— SPRINT OR OLYMPIC DISTANCE

According to coach Steven Truesdale, the following workout is designed to improve stamina, raise your lactate threshold, and increase power. This workout is basic training that all short- to medium-distance racers should do in order to develop core abilities requiring power in a 30-minute to 60-minute race course. Perform the workout on a flat time-trial course (with no traffic stops) or on a trainer.

Warm-up: Ride 15 minutes at approximately 90 RPM, at a very low intensity.

Workout: Ride five intervals of 5 minutes each at a moderately hard pace that you would only be able to sustain for 30 minutes. Recover fully at a moderate pace between intervals.

Cool-down: Ride for 15 to 20 minutes at an easy pace.

Subsequent workouts: Add 1 minute per week per interval, until you can maintain 5 intervals lasting 10 minutes at the same moderately hard pace as described previously.

HILLS

In his book, *Personal Best*, George Sheehan vividly describes a dogfight during a running race, a battle that pits him against one of his age-group competitors, as well as a third opponent: a hill.

> Just before the hill I pass him and go into second place in my age-group. It is a short-lived moment of triumph. The hill suddenly puts urgent demands on my body. . . . My legs are heavy and filled with pain. My breath comes in short gasps. I am bent over almost double. The battle shifts. It becomes me against me. My will in a duel with my mind and my body. A contest with that part of myself who wants to stop. (Sheehan 1989)

All of us, at one time or another, have come across hills like that one. Although I live in a part of the country that is relatively flat, I've always sought out opportunities to develop running power with a hilly course or leg strength with interval work on the bike. Whether interval bike workouts or running hills, power workouts can pay huge dividends to both mind and spirit.

Why run or bike hills? Besides the obvious cardiovascular benefits, there are significant strength-training benefits that can translate into pure power during a sprint to the finish line. Running or riding uphill is an excellent workout for major muscle groups that may typically be weak, such as hamstrings. Running downhill both increases coordination skills and strengthens vital quadriceps.

However, like any type of new training tool, hill workouts should be approached cautiously. Without a proper base, a safe course, and the right technique, hill running or riding may cause injuries such as shin splints, calf tears, and knee soreness. The following paragraphs present technique tips for keeping your hill workouts safe and effective.

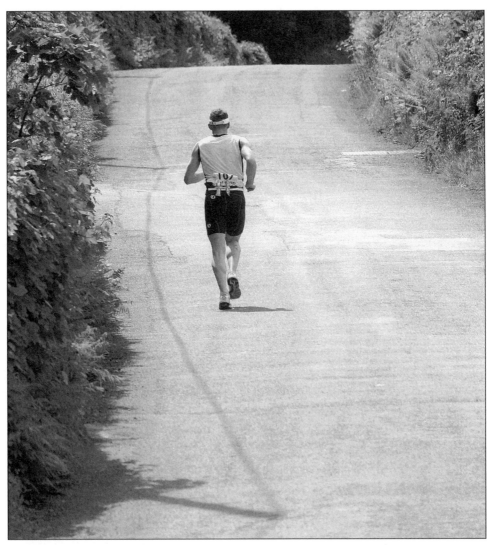

© Nigel Farrow

Hills offer both a personal challenge and an opportunity to increase power.

Cycling Hills

If you intend to ride a lot of hills or live in an area of the country where there is no avoiding them, the first thing you need to consider is upgrading your pedals to a clipless system. You will be able to ride much more efficiently uphill with pedal strokes that work through the entire 360-degree range of motion. Most noteworthy, clipless pedals provide an ability to pull up with each pedal stroke. One other note—don't let a poorly maintained bicycle hold you back; lube and clean the drivetrain and make sure your tires are inflated to the right pressure.

Climbing technique is important on the bike. Here are some quick tips:

- Find a gear that helps you establish a good rhythm; change it as frequently as you need to when you climb.
- Keep your upper body relaxed; avoid holding the handlebars in a death grip.
- Conserve energy—stay in your saddle and stand only when you need to stretch or on particularly steep grades.
- If you have to get off the saddle on steep grades, leverage power from your handlebars and rock back and forth.
- Don't forget to breathe; remember, stay relaxed.
- Set a pace that you think you can maintain throughout the climb.
- Keep your eyes peeled for potholes and obstacles; anticipate turns on fast downhills.

▶ SAMPLE CYCLING HILL WORKOUT

This workout, provided by Coach S.T., is designed to improve the function of your lactic and anaerobic systems, advance muscular development, increase stroke volume and blood lactate buffering, and boost stamina. According to Coach S.T., these workouts are best conducted after a base-training foundation has been built, with sufficient fitness for handling a much higher-intensity workout. Do this power workout on a course with one or more long hills.

Warm-up: Ride 15 minutes at approximately 90 RPM at a very low intensity.

Workout: Do four intervals—each interval is 2 minutes of high-intensity climbing while seated, followed by a very hard effort (an attack), riding out of the saddle for 30 seconds. Recover fully between intervals.

Cool-down: Ride at an easy pace for 15 to 20 minutes.

Running Hills

The first thing is to determine whether you are a better uphill or downhill runner. Are you always passed on a hilly course on the ascents, only to gain ground on the downhills? Or is your competition hurtling past you at warp speed while you shuffle down hills?

To be a good uphill *and* downhill runner, focus on your weakness so that you're a balanced hill runner. But keep in mind that running downhill requires less oxygen than running uphill. If you're not a good climber and you're in a race situation, you may want to concentrate on gaining ground on downhills.

Here are some quick technique tips for running uphill:

- Pace yourself based on the distance up the hill.
- Shorten your stride.
- Lean into the hill.
- Keep your arms low for better balance.
- Pump your arms (but don't exaggerate the motion).

When running downhill, follow these guidelines:

- Lengthen your stride.
- Don't put the brakes on (unless you have to).
- Keep your arms higher for better balance.
- Stay loose and avoid tightening up.

As you become more and more proficient at running both uphill and downhill on your favorite challenging trail or hilly road course, you'll quite likely find that your workouts on flat terrain seem like a breeze. Best of all, you'll be ready for the hilly triathlon running leg, and you'll have some extra power to outrun your age-group nemesis at your next race.

▶ SAMPLE HILL-RUNNING WORKOUT

Ideally, you want to perform this workout on a course that gives you 1 or 2 miles (1.6 or 3.2 kilometers) of flat terrain for a good warm-up. A course with multiple hills is best. If that isn't possible, you may have to use the one or two hills on your course over and over.

Warm-up: Run on flat terrain at an easy pace for 15 minutes.

Workout: As you approach the hills, gauge the steepness (grade) and distance and adjust your pace accordingly. Focus on maintaining a steady pace that you can keep throughout the climb. Use good hill-running form, leaning forward and using your arms for balance and momentum. As you hit the peak, recover with a slow jog or, if you have an immediate descent, run downhill with good form. Start by running only two hills and gradually work your way up to six by adding one more climb every 2 to 3 weeks.

Cool-down: Run at an easy pace for 15 to 20 minutes.

Structuring Your Hill Power Workouts

The easiest way to run or ride a power workout on hills is simply to find a course that presents these gravitational challenges throughout a medium distance, such as a 6-mile (9.7-kilometer) run or a 30-mile (48-kilometer) bike ride. Ideally, the hard work should begin after a proper warm-up of 1 or 2 miles (1.6 or 3.2 kilometers) for a run or 15 minutes for riding.

If such a course isn't available, try to find one or two decent-size hills in your locale. Even where I live, in the prairie fields of Illinois, there are hilly roads or other options for hill running, although you have to go out of your way to find them. Good places to look for great hill running are state parks or forest preserves. In this case, you may have to structure your workouts much like track intervals, using the lone hill or two as your hill repeat and doubling back to continue a series of repeats.

As with track workouts, you don't want to overdo the hills, especially if you have not done this type of training in a while. Whether you have a good hilly course nearby or have to seek out one or two hills and use them as repeats, start out at a modest pace and with no more than two climbs. Gradually add a climb every other week.

BRICKS

It's often said that triathlons all come down to the running. I disagree. Although you certainly have to be a good runner to be a competitive triathlete, you also have to come off the bike with legs that haven't been mangled beyond their running abilities. That's a lesson that many triathletes fail to learn. Although most triathlons finish with a run, it doesn't matter how good a runner you are if you don't adapt to running off the bike.

Brick workouts attempt to simulate two-thirds of triathlon conditions by combining two sports into one workout, such as swimming immediately followed by a bike ride or, more commonly, cycling followed by a run. Swim-to-bike bricks can help your transition to the bike if you are plagued by that loopy feeling in your legs off the swim. Here, however, we'll focus on a critical aspect of triathlon, the so-called T2 transition from bike to run.

Brick workouts not only help your body adapt to the rigors of transitioning from one sport to another but also give you a psychological edge. While others are fumbling out of the water or doing a death march on the run leg, you'll have a spring in your step and a smile on your face. Okay, maybe you won't feel that great, but with a regular dose of bricks you're sure to build yourself a successful triathlon season.

Workouts that simulate the transition from bike to run can be arduous and require a fair amount of commitment, so it's important to keep a few things in mind.

- Although bricks can be a part of your training on a regular basis, you may do well to focus on these demanding and time-consuming workouts for one to three months before an event, depending on your current conditioning and race goals.

- Because even the shortest of brick workouts involves two disciplines and a fair amount of gear preparation, you may want to plan these sessions for weekends or on days when you have more time. Be realistic about how much time you'll spend on your bike and on the run so that you can appropriately plan around your weekend obligations. You may also want to review the time-management tips in chapter 2 when planning your brick workouts.

- Bricks can help you hone your transitioning skills but only if you correctly simulate the T2 environment of a race. To do so, prepare a mock transition area set up as in a race and execute your T2 transition as quickly as possible. If you'll be doing a brick from your home, you can set up your transition area on a beach towel or blanket in the garage. Time your transitions and make it a goal to shave off five seconds each brick workout.

- Make sure you drink plenty of fluids—doing so will minimize the chances of cramping during the bike-to-run transition.

Sample Brick Workouts

Many possibilities for bike-run brick workouts exist, and how you structure them will depend not only on the race distance you are training for but also on which of the two you consider to be your weaker sport. The first two sample brick workouts that follow will help you strengthen your weakest discipline, and the third will help you improve your overall performance in both race legs.

▶ BIKE-EMPHASIS BRICK WORKOUT

If you want to get a good idea of how you will feel in a race coming off the saddle, a bike-emphasis brick will give you just that. In fact, the bike portion will be almost as demanding as any single workout you'll do, and the run portion of the brick is designed to accustom the legs to running at an easy transitional pace for a relatively short distance.

Bike distance: The bike portion of your brick can be anywhere from 60 to 90 percent of the actual race distance. For example, if you're training for an Ironman, your ride can be between 67 and 100 miles (108 and 161 kilometers). If you're training for an Olympic-distance race, ride somewhere between 15 and 22 miles (24 and 35 kilometers).

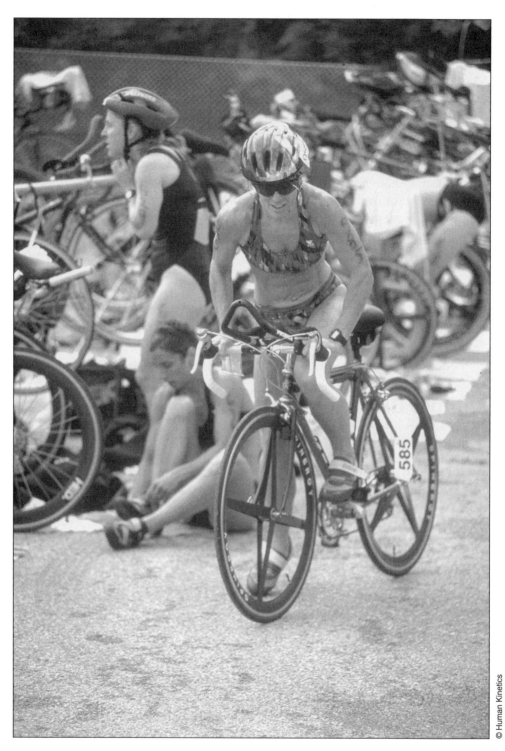

Brick workouts ensure smooth transitions on race day, giving you an edge over the competition.

Bike intensity: This should be a fairly difficult ride, with a pace and intensity of close to 80 percent of your race pace. If there are hills in your target race, try to ride a course with similar terrain.

Transition 2 (T2): Your transition off the bike should mimic your race, so make it quick and smooth.

Run distance: The run portion of this brick should be only 25 percent of your actual race leg distance—for example, 6.5 miles for an Ironman or about a 5K for a half-Ironman distance.

Run intensity: Your pace and intensity should mimic that of an easy cooldown, particularly if you have had trouble running off the bike in the past. Remember, the goal here is to progressively accustom yourself to running off a pretty intense bike leg; it is not designed for race-pace running.

▶ RUN-EMPHASIS BRICK WORKOUT

If running is what you need to work on the most, a bike-to-run brick with heavy emphasis on the running can improve your confidence on race day. In addition, if you are planning a long run, adding a relatively easy bike ride can act as a fantastic warm-up.

Bike distance: If you are training for an Ironman or half-Ironman, plan to ride anywhere from 20 to 40 percent of your race's bike distance. For an Olympic- or sprint-distance race, ride 7 to 10 miles (11 to 16 kilometers).

Bike intensity: Your ride should be at an easy to moderate intensity, about 50 to 60 percent of race pace. It's OK to ride hills, but pace yourself accordingly and work on good hill-climbing technique as opposed to mashing big gears or expending lots of energy.

T2: Execute a quick transition and establish a rhythm and tempo in the first few miles or kilometers that you can maintain for the entire course.

Run distance: Your run leg should consist of 70 to 90 percent of your actual race distance. For example, a half-Ironman brick session would include a 9- to 12-mile (15- to 19-kilometer) run.

Run intensity: Run at an intensity that is about 80 percent of your race pace. If there will be hills on the race course, make them a part of your run for this brick workout.

▶ TIME-TRIAL BRICK

A time-trial brick can also be considered a race simulation workout and can be structured according to the following guidelines (with regard to course and conditions). It is a high-intensity workout, and you should perform it only periodically in the few months before a race. It mimics the intensity of a time trial in which you expend as much energy as possible throughout the entire distance; however, I recommend that you notch it down to about 80 percent of your race pace in order to build your fitness toward actual race-pace performance over time.

Bike distance: Ride 40 to 50 percent of your actual race for Ironman or half-Ironman distances. Olympic- and sprint-distance triathletes should ride 7 to 10 miles (11 to 16 kilometers).

Bike intensity: Ride at 80 percent of race pace on a course that mimics the topography of your race.

T2: Make it a speedy transition. Hit the ground running off the saddle and settle into your pace right away.

Run distance: Run 50 percent of your actual race distance.

Run intensity: Run at 80 percent of race pace on a course that mimics the event.

Brick Variations

You can choose from many different possibilities for structuring bricks, which makes designing these workouts fun, challenging, and a great strategy for customizing your training to fit your individual goals. For example, bring your running shoes to your next weekend century ride and go out for an easy 3-mile (4.8-kilometer) cool-down (you'll raise some eyebrows in the parking lot). Or you can ride your bike to the starting line of your favorite 10K (you'll also raise some eyebrows, but you'll surely lose that notoriety in the first few miles). Combining events like a century ride or organized run with another discipline is a great time-saver and motivating short-term goal, helping you effectively design a brick workout with a set course, time, and date.

RACE SIMULATIONS

Have you ever stood at the starting line of a race and had no idea what to expect? All of us are probably guilty at one time or another of being underprepared for the specific race conditions that lie before us as we anticipate the starting gun. It takes courage and mental toughness to embrace the unknown in a race we've never done before, but it's also better to be prepared than not.

Bricks provide a great way to simulate the general conditions of going from your bike to a run, but race simulation workouts go a step further and focus on an essential element of performance—being prepared for the conditions and the course. There are many possible ways to simulate a race. Here are some tips to help you lay the groundwork for an effective simulation.

• **Research the course.** The first step in attempting to simulate the race that you are training for is to research what challenges the course will present. There are several ways to do this, but most of the information you need can be obtained on the Internet. Many triathlon organizers present this information on their Web sites. If they don't, contact the race officials and see whether you can get as much detailed information as possible. Some races may even offer topographical maps or sample training workouts based on the course.

• **Research the conditions.** For races in climates different from your own, it's important to get as much information as you can on what to expect when you toe the line. Sources of possible information include weather sites, the race Web site, *Farmer's Almanac,* and fellow competitors who have raced the event.

• **Take advantage of weather opportunities.** Do you live in one of the northern states and find yourself training in the middle of winter for a warm-weather race on the West Coast? Sometimes it's simply impossible to adequately prepare for certain race conditions, such as heat, humidity, wind, rain, and so forth. However, if the opportunity presents itself, you should always try to perform a high-intensity workout, long ride, long run, or brick on a day when the weather mirrors the race conditions you'll be facing.

• **Prepare for swim conditions.** The swim leg of a triathlon is perhaps one of its most distinguishing characteristics—every one is different, often in very big ways. For example, the swim portion of the Accenture Chicago Triathlon is perhaps one of the most harrowing. Here thousands of swimmers jump into Lake Michigan with arms and legs flailing, and at times it may seem as if they're all swimming on your back. If you'll be up against a crowded swim, perhaps one of the best race simulations you can do is swimming in open water with a few training partners alongside you to help you become accustomed to a crowd (and the occasional kick in the face). Better yet, open-water swim events are a great way to simulate hectic conditions.

▶ SAMPLE RACE SIMULATION WORKOUT (IRONMAN DISTANCE)

This brick simulation workout, recommended by coach Steven Truesdale, is best done on alternating weekends at least one month before your Ironman-distance race. Find a 3-hour bike ride route that allows long, steady efforts in the saddle and simulates your race route to some degree. Set up a mock transition zone in your garage with your running gear, a towel, and food and fluid supplies, just as you would at a race. For the run portion, find a loop or out-and-back route that is relatively flat but that may have some short hills in it. The total workout times can be extended, from 3 hours at first up to 5 or more hours as you get closer to the end of your peak training period. Your longest time should be the last brick you do before you settle into your taper. After this workout, make sure you get a solid recovery over the next 24 hours.

Warm-up: Ride at a slow and easy pace for 45 to 60 minutes at approximately 90 RPM.

Workout stage 1: Maintain a steady 90 to 120 minutes at your race pace. Be careful not to exceed your maximum steady state effort; back off if you have to for hills.

Workout stage 2: Transition quickly as you would on race day, and take off on foot for a moderate-length run of 60 to 120 minutes.

Cool-down: Walk for about 10 minutes after your run to help your legs and body recover.

WEAKNESSES

Almost any triathlete, whether beginner or Ironman veteran, is sure to agree on one training principle—focusing on your weakest sport during training will yield significant performance returns. Yet, despite the general agreement on the benefits of shoring up your weakness, there seems to be a prevalence of triathletes who don't do it.

Why do so many triathletes avoid a training emphasis on their weakest sport? I suppose it's human nature to take the path of least resistance. I suspect it's also natural to avoid an activity that seems more difficult in comparison with the other two.

For example, I've known several triathletes through the years who have consistently had a difficult time riding on roads—fearing accidents, being uncomfortable with speed, or balking at more than an hour in the saddle. Of course, perhaps the most common example is the triathlete who fears deep water and thus never gains a high level of proficiency in swimming, let alone open-water navigation. Triathletes who don't come from a running background can often find pounding the pavement torturous.

But if you are committed to gaining ground on your triathlon race times, there is no better 80/20 activity than any workout that forces you to focus on your weakest link. We've already outlined a couple of brick workouts with a greater emphasis on running or cycling, which are terrific ways to really work on a weakness. But don't stop there. Really commit to and plan out workouts in your training calendar that consistently push you to work on the one or two disciplines that challenge you the most, both physically and mentally. If you do so, you'll find that these select, targeted workouts definitely yield the biggest returns on your race performances—that's really the whole concept behind 80/20 workouts.

It may be a bitter pill to swallow, but working on the weakest of the three disciplines need not be torture. You must develop a mindset that you will gradually make inroads with your weak sport; nothing is going to happen overnight. Here are a few tips for tackling your weakness:

• **Increase your weakness proportion.** If you divide your training time per week into pie slices, which percentage are you allocating to working on your weakest sport? If your weakness is cycling and you spend 50 percent of your time running, 30 percent of your time swimming, and only 20 percent of your time on the saddle, chances are you'll make very few cycling gains at your next race. When you do your weekly planning, bump up the percentage of time you spend on your weakest sport so that it is at least proportional to (or even better, more than) the other two disciplines.

• **Find training partners for mentoring.** Other than swim drills, there is no better way to gain some ground on your weakest sport than to find a training partner who will motivate you and push you to train harder, faster, or farther. Ideally, you can find a training partner who can be your guiding light in one sport, whereas you can be the motivator in another.

• **Get the right gear.** Sometimes your unwillingness to get on the bike or go out for a run has more to do with your gear than with anything else. If you are uncomfortable on your bike or if your feet hurt in your running shoes, maybe a trip to the bike shop or specialty running store is all you need to make working on your weak link more enjoyable.

• **Get in a groove.** When I first learned to swim properly in my early 20s, I dreaded the thought of going to the pool. But I committed to working on it at least three times a week, sometimes four or five. After a few months, the mental dynamic of my pool workouts changed. It started to become something I actually enjoyed—the cool sensation of the water, the pleasure of moving my body through the water, and the soothing tiredness of a good workout without the aches and pains from pounding the pavement or mashing gears. Although it may be difficult at first to tackle working on your weakness consistently with a positive mental attitude, you'll most likely find that soon you start looking forward to it.

PART III

Race Programs

Now that you have a good idea of the types of workouts you can incorporate into your training and have read about ways you can fit them all into your busy life, this section provides sample training plans for each of the four major triathlon distances. All the planning and log pages you need to get everything down on paper are here in an easy-to-use format.

CHAPTER 8

Sprint Training

T he sprint distance is the most common distance for the novice triathlete, but it can also be a challenging race for anybody looking to go
fast in a relatively short period. For the beginner, it's the ideal distance
for getting your feet wet.

Whereas the image of the triathlon among the worldwide media may be
more in line with the gruel-a-thon picture painted at the Ironman Champi-
onships in Hawaii, the sprint distance is fast becoming the most popular
choice for those with limited time or the desire to lead a more balanced
lifestyle. And although anybody with good time-management skills can
train for even the longer distances and still maintain a balanced life, it sure
is easier when your weekly training totals need not exceed 10 hours.

Sprint-distance triathlons require the least amount of time commitment
on your part. That doesn't mean you won't be challenged, particularly if
you are weak in one or more of the three disciplines. Also, the amount of
your effort and your commitment to training depend on whether you are
doing your first triathlon, using the race as a training event, or going for
broke to place in your age-group (or even win).

The sprint-distance workouts that follow are an example of what typical
training may encompass for this length of triathlon. They are intended as
snapshots of sprint-distance training, not the definitive word on how to
train, because there is no definitive word. When planning your training
for maximum effectiveness, always modify any sample plan or template,
including the ones in this book, to suit your individual goals. Part of the
fun and excitement of planning and executing your training is the creative
element. Much of triathlon training theory is backed by science, but it's as
much an art as a science when you start applying these theories to your
individual goals, unique body, and mental attitude. If you already have
a good feel for your training, you may find elements in sample workouts
presented here that you'll want to incorporate into your existing plan.

As with all formulaic training schedules, you should customize your sprint-distance training to suit these conditions:

- Current fitness level
- Goals
- Strengths
- Weaknesses
- Technical weaknesses (such as poor swimming technique)
- Injuries or other limitations
- Special disabilities
- Topography of the race course
- Any other conditions of the race course

The sample workout in table 8.1 includes a variety of approaches to training, such as key workouts, heart rate workouts, and 80/20 workouts. In addition, I've included both time-based workouts and distance-based training—use whatever approach you feel most comfortable with.

Personally, I prefer time-based workouts, especially early in a training cycle. Instead of being overly preoccupied with distance, focusing on time allows you to complete the training at your most appropriate pace instead of pushing yourself too hard to finish a 3-mile (4.8-kilometer) run in a so-called respectable time.

The eight-week matrix in this chapter also features a significant chunk of training on weekends, when you probably have more time. If your schedule is not typical (for example, a fireman's schedule might consist of consecutive 24-hour work days followed by several days off), simply transfer the weekend workouts shown here to days that are best suited for you. Just make sure to take your recovery day or your day off immediately after high-intensity, demanding efforts.

You'll notice that Mondays are typically a recovery day or day off. I'm a big believer in giving yourself at least one day of rest. Because hard workouts are usually done on the weekends, Mondays are well suited for recovery.

With any formula, you need to personalize the tapering period to your own situation. Here are some considerations for determining your ideal tapering schedule:

- Your age
- Your rate of recovery from a workout
- Your intensity and volume of training in the month before the race
- Your travel time to a distant race
- Your mental state (if you're burned out on training, maybe you need a little more tapering)

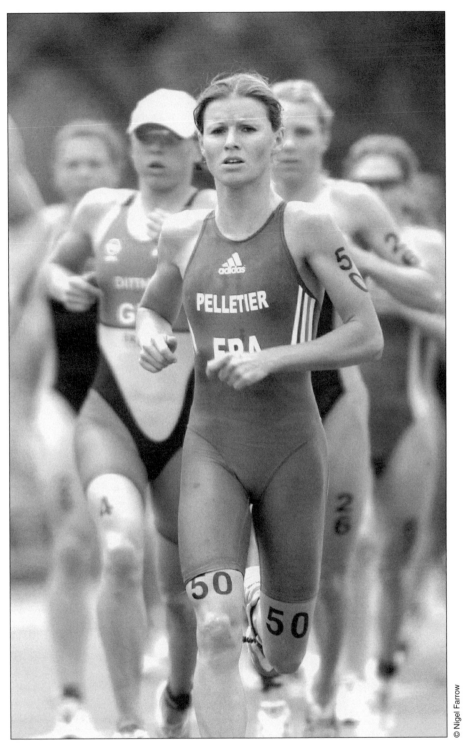

While sprint-distance races don't require as much time commitment or training as other distances, they are still very challenging.

Table 8.1 Training Snapshot for a Sprint-Distance Triathlon

	Monday	Tuesday	Wednesday
Week 1	(swim) (KEY): Brainwork sample workout on p. 72	(bike) (HR): 7 mi (11K) in recovery and endurance zone	(swim): Drills (run): 15 min easy walk or run (optional)
Week 2	Recovery day (off)	(swim) (KEY): Race simulation sample workout on p. 73, distance decreased to 900 m	(bike) (HR): 7 mi (11K) in recovery and endurance zone
Week 3	Recovery day (off)	(swim) (KEY): Hard-easy-hard sample workout on p. 74	(bike): 8 mi (13K) easy spinning at 90 RPM or higher
Week 4	Recovery day (off)	(swim) (KEY): Countdown sample workout on p. 74, decrease to 750 m swim as a 350, 250, 100, 50	(bike): 10 mi (16K) easy spinning at 90 RPM or higher
Week 5	Recovery day (off)	(swim) (80/20): Race simulation swim in supervised open water for 15 min; or 20 min swim in pool, practicing navigational sighting skills	(bike): 12 mi (19K) easy spinning at 90 RPM or higher
Week 6	Recovery day (off)	(swim) (KEY): Hold a pace sample workout on p. 74, modify to 10 x 25 m with 10 sec rest	(bike): 10 mi (16K) at moderate pace with two 1 mi (1.6K) race pace efforts in the middle miles
Week 7	Recovery day (off)	(swim) (KEY): Technique golf sample workout on p. 73, 10 x 25 m with 15-30 sec rest	(bike): Group ride of 10-15 mi (16-24K)
Week 8	Recovery day (off)	(swim) (KEY): Sustainable pace sample workout on p. 73, with race distance divided into two parts (2 x 375 m)	(run) (interval): 1 mi (1.6K) easy warm-up; 2-4 x .25 mi (0.4K), resting 30-60 sec between intervals; 1 mi (1.6K) cool-down

Note: Although it is not always specified here, always warm up and cool down properly with an easy effort. When distance or time isn't specified, use your own discretion for completing the workout in a distance that's right for your current fitness and ability levels. Always create your own plan based on your current training stage and individual goals.

Thursday	Friday	Saturday	Sunday
(swim): 500 m easy (bike): 20 min easy	(run): 15 min easy run	(bike): 7 mi (11K) easy spinning at 90 RPM or higher	(run) (KEY): 20 min easy
(run): 20 min walk or run (swim): Drills	(swim): 500 m easy	(bike): 8 mi (13K) easy spinning at 90 RPM or higher	(run) (HR): 20 min in recovery and endurance zone
(run): 20 min easy	(swim): Drills	(bike) (HR): 7 mi (11K) in recovery and endurance zone	(run) (KEY): 20 min run; first 15 min easy with 5 min tempo run at the end
(run): 15 min easy	(swim): Drills	(bike) (KEY): Pedaling efficiency workout on p. 76	(run) (HR): 25 min easy run in recovery and endurance zone
(run) (KEY): 15 min tempo run or HR run in aerobic and tempo zone	(swim): 500 m easy, followed by drills	(bike) (KEY): 8 mi (13K) hilly course at moderate pace with recovery on downhills	(run) (HR): 25 min easy run in recovery and endurance zone
(run): Group run of 3-5 mi (4.8-8K) at conversational pace, or 20 min easy run	(swim): 750 m easy; followed by drills	(bike): 8 mi (13K) easy spinning at 90 RPM or higher	(bike)/(run) brick (80/20) (bike): 10 mi (16K) at a moderate pace or in the aerobic and tempo zone (run): 15 min easy
(run): 10 min easy followed by 5 min at near race pace, 5 min easy cool-down	(swim): 700 m easy, followed by drills	(bike) (HR): Heart rate workout on p. 76	(run) (HR): 3 mi (4.8K) in aerobic and tempo zone
(swim): 500 m followed by drills	(run): 15 min easy	(bike) (HR): 12 mi (19K) in aerobic and tempo zone	(run): 25 min easy

Depending on these considerations, you can choose to do a three-day taper or a weeklong one (see the following lists). The tables show the total amount of time you should spend training. The charts don't specify exactly how you should be training, so use some common sense. Divide the disciplines proportionally according to what you've been doing.

However, if you feel overtrained or on the brink of injury, feel free to skew the training toward the sport that is least strenuous for you. For example, if you are experiencing some knee soreness from running too much or too hard, do more easy swimming in the weeks before your event, allowing your body to recover in time for the race.

Half-Week Taper for Sprint-Distance Triathlon

Day 1	20 min
Day 2	15 min
Day 3	Complete rest
Day 4	Race day

One-Week Taper for Sprint-Distance Triathlon

Day 1	30 min
Day 2	Complete rest
Day 3	25 min
Day 4	20 min
Day 5	15 min
Day 6	Complete rest
Day 7	Race day

CHAPTER 9

Olympic Training

The Olympic distance is the middle ground of triathlon races. It is perhaps too challenging for the beginner, but it is ideal for those who seek a moderate amount of training commitment or a stepping-stone for the longer distances.

Many novice triathletes do feel comfortable tackling this distance, particularly those who have a solid background in one or more of the three disciplines. If you are a beginner and are considering an Olympic distance race, just be sure it's an event with a relatively small number of participants (in the hundreds, as opposed to the thousands). Large races are fun, but I wouldn't recommend one as your first tri-event.

If you're among the triathletes who start with a sprint-distance triathlon and work their way up to the Olympic distance and beyond, consider a couple of unique factors. Since the distances are double that of the sprint, your training will of course increase. Will it double? Not always. The reason is simple—to do a sprint-distance triathlon (perhaps your first) you probably had a big learning curve in terms of skills and knowledge, and you most likely had to focus a fair amount of your workout time on base training. You'll carry over some of these credits, so to speak, if you choose to graduate to Olympic distance.

The Olympic distance also forces you to think more about pace. It challenges you to maintain an optimum pace that you can execute throughout three disciplines at this particular distance, the same way you would run at a slower pace during a 10K than you would in a 5K. Whereas you may have had the luxury of pushing the limits at times during a sprint triathlon, doing so at this distance and longer can leave you unable to recover and perform in the latter half of a race.

As you tackle this distance and longer, maintaining a steady pace and intensity throughout a race is an increasingly important factor in both your training and triathlon execution. Bricks in particular are helpful in this regard, especially workouts like the race simulation brick detailed in chapter 7.

Olympic-distance triathlons require a moderate time commitment on your part, usually anywhere from 10 to 15 hours a week, depending on your goals. The Olympic-distance workouts shown here are meant to be an example of what typical training may encompass for this event, not the definitive word.

To individualize your Olympic-distance training, take into account the following factors:

- Current fitness level
- Goals
- Strengths
- Weaknesses
- Technical weaknesses (such as poor swimming technique)
- Injuries or other limitations
- Special disabilities
- Topography of the race course
- Any other conditions of the race course

The sample workouts include a variety of approaches: key workouts, heart rate training, and 80/20 workouts. Settle on your most effective method or use a variety to achieve your goals. In addition, I've included both time-based workouts and distance-based training—use whatever approach you feel most comfortable with. As in all the training grids, Mondays are typically a recovery day or day off. In my opinion, Mondays are the ideal day to recover from hard weekend workouts and refresh yourself for the training ahead.

Once again, you need to customize any regimen for your situation. Here are some considerations for determining your ideal tapering schedule:

- Your age
- Your rate of recovery from a workout
- Your intensity and volume of training in the month before the race
- Your travel time to a distant race
- Your mental state (if you're burned out on training, maybe you need a little more tapering)

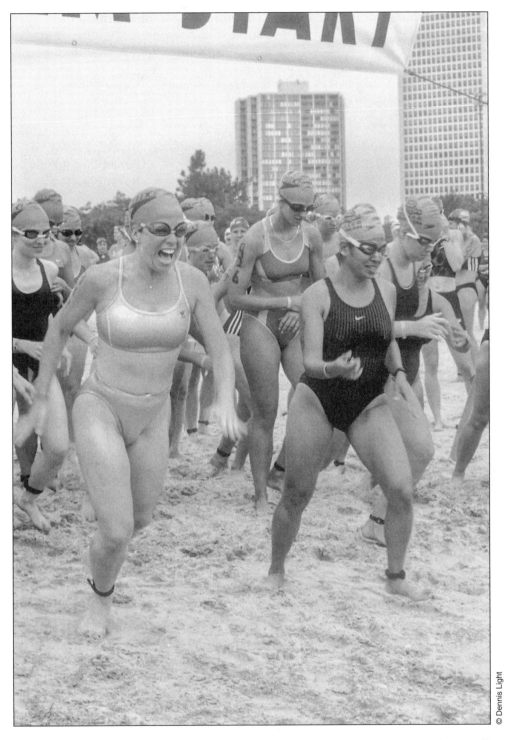

Beginning Olympic-distance triathletes should consider competing in races with a small number of competitors, which can be just as fun as larger races.

Table 9.1 Training Snapshot for an Olympic-Distance Triathlon

	Monday	Tuesday	Wednesday
Week 1	(KEY): Brainwork p. 72, distance modified to 1500 m	(HR): 15 mi (24K) in recovery and endurance zone	: 20 min easy
Week 2	Recovery day (off)	(KEY): Race simulation on p. 73 1500 m	(HR): 15 mi (24K) in recovery and endurance zone
Week 3	Recovery day (off)	(KEY): Technique golf sample workout on p. 73, modified to 8 x 25 m	: 15 mi (24K) easy spinning at 90 RPM or higher
Week 4	Recovery day (off)	(KEY): Sustainable pace sample workout on p. 73, modified to 2 x 750 m	: 20 mi (32K) easy spinning at 90 RPM or higher
Week 5	Recovery day (off)	(80/20): Race simulation swim of 25 min in supervised open water; or 30 min swim in pool, practicing navigational sighting skills	: 15 mi (24K) easy spinning at 90 RPM or higher
Week 6	Recovery day (off)	(KEY): Hold a pace workout on p. 74, 10 x 25 m with 10 sec rest at fast, even pace	: 20 mi (32K) at a moderate pace with 5 x 1 mi (1.6K) race pace efforts in the middle and 5 min recovery between efforts
Week 7	Recovery day (off)	(KEY): Countdown sample workout on p. 74, modified to 1500 m swim as a 500, 400, 300, 200, 100	: Group ride of 20-25 mi (32-40K)
Week 8	Recovery day (off)	(KEY): Hard-easy-hard sample workout on p. 74	(interval): 1 mi (1.6K) easy warm-up; 3-4 x .25 mi (0.4K), 1-2 x .50 mi (0.8K), resting 30-60 sec between intervals; 1 mi cool-down

Note: Although it is not always specified here, always warm up and cool down properly with an easy effort. When distance or time isn't specified, use your own discretion for completing the workout in a distance that's right for your current fitness and ability levels. Always create your own plan based on your current training stage and individual goals.

Thursday	Friday	Saturday	Sunday
: 1000 m easy : 30 min spinning at 90 RPM or higher	: Drills	: 15 mi (24K) easy spinning at 90 RPM or higher	(KEY): 30 min easy with fartlek surges at 5K race pace lasting 10-60 sec in the middle miles
: 30 min easy run : Drills	: 1000 m easy	: 20 mi (32K) easy spinning at 90 RPM or higher	(HR): 40 min run in recovery and endurance zone
: 35 min easy run	: Drills	(HR): 20 mi (32K) in recovery and endurance base zone	(KEY): 45 min run—15 min easy, 15 min tempo run, 15 min easy cool-down
: 30 min easy run	: Drills	(KEY): 60-90 minute speed workout, as described on p. 78	(HR): 50 min easy run in recovery and endurance zone
(KEY): 30 min tempo run or HR run in aerobic and tempo zone	: 1000 m easy, followed by drills	(KEY): 15 mi (24K) hilly bike course at moderate pace with recovery on downhills	(HR): 45 min easy run in recovery and endurance zone
: Group run of 5 mi (8K) at conversational pace, or run 40 min easy	: 1500 m easy, followed by drills	: 10 mi (16K) easy spinning at 90 RPM or higher	/ brick (80/20) : 20 mi (32K) at a moderate pace or in the aerobic and tempo zone : 30 min easy
: 20 min easy run followed by 5 min at near race pace, 5 min easy cool-down	: 1200 m easy, followed by drills	(HR): Heart rate sample workout on p. 76	(HR): 5 mi (8K) in aerobic and tempo zone
: 1200 m followed by drills	: 30 min easy	(HR): 25 mi (40K) in aerobic and tempo zone	: 1 hr easy, conversational pace

With an Olympic-distance event, you should consider a full week tapering period. See the following list for the total amount of time you should spend training. Divide the disciplines into the same proportions you've been doing or, if you'd like a little more recovery, focus on swimming drills and easy bikes and runs. Avoid any high-intensity training, such as track intervals or a very hilly course.

One-Week Taper for Olympic-Distance Triathlon

Day 1	45 min
Day 2	Complete rest
Day 3	40 min
Day 4	30 min
Day 5	20 min
Day 6	Complete rest
Day 7	Race day

CHAPTER 10

Half-Ironman Training

I must admit it: The half-Ironman is my favorite. In my view, it is the ideal triathlon distance. Why? Because it is demanding enough in both training and execution to give you a real feeling of accomplishment and happy exhaustion at the finish line, while not completely dominating your life the way the full Ironman distance might do. Although any triathlon can result in the same good feelings, depending on the individual, for me the half-Ironman is just right—not too short, not too long. I have raced this distance the most in my decade and a half of competing, an average of four a year, with a few shorter races thrown in for good measure.

If you're stepping up from a shorter distance, you'll quickly find that half-Ironman races require a significant amount of training time, especially to ensure that you'll be prepared for the cycling leg. Training time on the bike usually clocks in with the most hours (for any triathlon distance). For half-Ironman races, your long weekend rides might last anywhere from three to four hours in the saddle. Add a run after that for the occasional brick session, and you can see how easy it is for such training to eat up a good chunk of your day. Provided you're up to the task, it can be some of the most personally rewarding training you'll undertake.

We all know of hardy, stoic souls who enjoy training by themselves, but the half-Ironman is a race distance best tackled with a training partner. You need a compadre on your long bike rides and runs, and not just for passing the time with idle chitchat. A training partner for those long stretches on the road is simply safer than riding or running alone. You should always prepare yourself for contingencies and emergencies on a long bike ride (spare tubes, tire levers, air pump, first-aid kit, enough fluids, mobile phone), but with a fellow cyclist, you greatly improve your odds of staying safe while sharing the road with automobile traffic.

If you don't have a regular training partner, look for opportunities to ride in a group, such as a local bike shop ride or the weekend organized rides put on by cycling clubs in your area. Running clubs also host weekly runs on safe routes.

Another consideration if you're advancing to this demanding distance is upgrading your triathlon gear. With long hours in the saddle, it becomes even more important to have clothes that fit you well, a bicycle that is comfortable and is the right size for your body, and clipless pedals and shoes that make you more efficient (if you've been shopping the mass sporting goods chains for bike equipment, you may want to visit your local specialty cycling shop right about now). Also, make sure that your swimming goggles are comfortable and leakproof, and that your running shoes have enough cushioning left in them for the long runs you'll be doing (I generally buy a new pair every three to six months, a good rule of thumb for anybody running consistently). Half-Ironman training increases the stress on all your triathlon equipment enough that shortfalls become fairly evident over time, so take a good hard look at your current gear to determine whether you need to upgrade.

Half-Ironman triathlons require a significant commitment. This level of training dedication is not for everyone; keep in mind that you'll be splashing, mashing, and dashing anywhere from 15 hours a week at a minimum to upward of 25 or 30 hours a week for those chasing high-level performance.

As with all the workouts in this book, the half-Ironman workouts shown here are meant to give you a snapshot of what training might take for this event.

To individualize your half-Ironman distance training, take into account the following factors:

- Current fitness level
- Goals
- Strengths
- Weaknesses
- Technical weaknesses (such as poor swimming technique)
- Injuries or other limitations
- Special disabilities
- Topography of the race course
- Any other conditions of the race course

The sample workouts here include a variety of approaches to training: key workouts, heart rate training, and 80/20 workouts. Determine your most effective approach or use a variety to achieve your goals. You'll notice that both time-based workouts and distance-based training are shown on the workout charts—use whichever you feel most comfortable with.

As you can see, the training matrix usually gives you a day off or a recovery workout on Mondays. Because most of your hard or long workouts occur on the weekend, Monday is well suited for taking it easy or doing a low-intensity recovery workout of your choosing (it could even be bowling or pool).

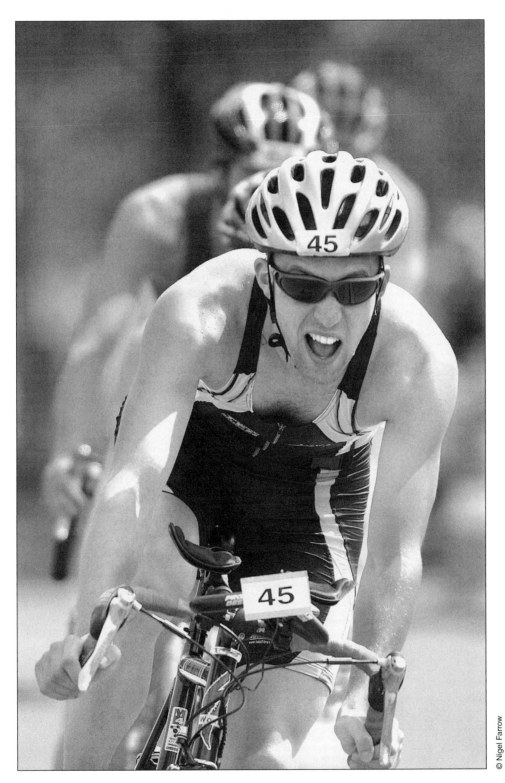

The half-Ironman distance requires a significant amount of time and intensity in both training and racing.

Table 10.1   Training Snapshot for a Half-Ironman Distance Triathlon

	Monday	Tuesday	Wednesday
Week 1	(KEY): Brainwork workout on p. 72, distance modified to 1900 m	(HR): 25 mi (40K) in recovery and endurance zone	: 40 min easy run
Week 2	Recovery day (off)	(KEY): Race simulation workout on p. 73, distance modified to 1900 m	(HR): 30 mi (48K) in recovery and endurance zone
Week 3	Recovery day (off)	(KEY): Technique golf workout on p. 73	: 30 mi (48K) easy spinning at 90 RPM or higher
Week 4	Recovery day (off)	(KEY): Sustainable pace workout on p. 73, distance modified to 2 x 950 m	: 40 mi (64K) easy spinning at 90 RPM or higher
Week 5	Recovery day (off)	(80/20): Race simulation swim in supervised open water for 50 min; or 45 min swim in pool, practicing navigational sighting skills	: 30 mi (48K) easy spinning at 90 RPM or higher
Week 6	Recovery day (off)	(KEY): Hold a pace workout on p. 74, distance modified to 10 x 75 m	: 40 mi (64K) at a moderate pace with 6 x 1 mi race pace efforts in the middle, 5 min recovery between efforts
Week 7	Recovery day (off)	(KEY): Countdown workout on p. 74	: Group ride of 40-50 mi (64-80K)
Week 8	Recovery day (off)	(KEY): Hard-easy-hard workout, distance modified to 4 x 75 m fast speed, 2 x 75 m very easy, and 4 x 75 m fast speed, all on 20-30 sec rest	(HR): 8 mi (13K) in aerobic and tempo zone

Note: Although it is not always specified here, always warm up and cool down properly with an easy effort. When distance or time isn't specified, use your own discretion for completing the workout in a distance that's right for your current fitness and ability levels. Always create your own plan based on your current training stage and individual goals.

Thursday	Friday	Saturday	Sunday
[swim]: 1500 m easy [bike]: 60 min spinning at 90 RPM or higher	[swim]: Drills	[bike]: 35 mi (56K) easy spinning at 90 RPM or higher	[run]: 1 hr easy
[run]: 45 min easy [swim]: Drills	[swim]: 1800 m easy	[bike]: 40 mi (64K) easy spinning at 90 RPM or higher [swim]: Drills	[run] (HR): 1 hr run in recovery and endurance zone
[run]: 45 min easy run, throwing in some fartlek surges in the middle miles if you feel good	[swim]: Drills	[bike] (HR): 40 mi (64K) in recovery and endurance zone [swim]: 6 x 75 m at moderate pace concentrating on form; 30 sec rest between intervals	[run] (KEY): 1 hr run—20 min easy, 20 min tempo run, 20 min easy cool-down
[run]: 45 min easy run	[swim]: Drills	[bike] (KEY): Speed workout on p. 78 [swim]: 1800 m easy	[run] (HR): 1 hr easy run at recovery and endurance zone
[run] (KEY): 45 min tempo run or HR run in aerobic and tempo zone	[swim]: 1800 m easy, followed by drills	[bike] (KEY): 30 mi (48K) hilly bike course at moderate pace with recovery on downhills	[run] (HR): 70 min easy run at recovery and endurance base zone [swim]: Drills
[run]: Group run of 6-8 mi (9.7-13K) at conversational pace, or 45 min easy run [swim]: Drills	[swim]: 2000 m easy, followed by drills	[bike]: 25 mi (40K) easy spinning at 90 RPM or higher	[bike]/[run] brick (80/20) [bike]: 40 mi (64K) at a moderate pace or in the aerobic and tempo zone [run]: 1 hr easy
[run] (intervals): 1 mi (1.6K) easy warm-up; 2 x .25 mi, 3 x .50 mi, 2 x .25 mi, resting 1 min between intervals; 1 mi (1.6K) easy cool-down	[swim]: 2000 m easy, followed by drills	[bike] (HR): 40 mi (64K) in aerobic and tempo zone	[run] (HR): 10 mi (16K) in aerobic and tempo zone [swim]: Drills
[swim]: 2000 m followed by drills	[run]: 45 min easy	[bike] (HR): 50 mi (80K) in aerobic and tempo zone	[run]: 90 min easy, conversational pace [swim]: Drills

As with any formula, customize your training to suit your uniqueness. The following are some considerations for determining your ideal tapering schedule:

- Your age
- Your rate of recovery from a workout
- Your intensity and volume of training in the month before the race
- Your travel time to a distant race
- Your mental state (if you're burned out on training, maybe you need a little more tapering)

With a half-Ironman distance event, you should consider a 10-day tapering schedule. The following list indicates the total amount of time you should spend training. Simply divide the disciplines into the same proportions that you've been doing, or if you'd like a little more recovery, focus on swimming drills and easy rides and runs. Avoid any high-intensity training, such as track intervals, especially during the last week before your event.

Ten-Day Half-Ironman Taper

Day 1	60 min
Day 2	Complete rest
Day 3	45 min
Day 4	40 min
Day 5	40 min
Day 6	Complete rest
Day 7	30 min
Day 8	20 min
Day 9	Complete rest
Day 10	Race day

CHAPTER 11

Ironman Training

In my circle of friends who participate in endurance sports such as marathons and triathlons, we have a saying: Never mess with a marathon. And you definitely never, ever want to mess with an Ironman. The connotation is that whereas some experienced athletes may be able to get away with minimal preparation for short- or medium-distance events, the Ironman distance race is something you must go into with a level of preparation sufficient to ensure a safe and relatively pain-free race.

But don't let the higher level scare you if you feel you are prepared to meet this challenge. Although the Ironman distance is demanding, good time management and a healthy dose of moderation in all things can help ensure that your training is both fun and balanced. Without moderation in your training, your life can definitely be turned upside down. So pay special attention to other key areas of your life (work, your marriage, etc.) that could potentially suffer if you're overdoing things a bit. Of course, symptoms of overtraining will also indicate a lack of moderation.

Although this distance has been tackled in less time by veteran triathletes with a solid fitness foundation in all three sports, a training plan that spans a year is ideal (assuming you are not a novice, in which case an Ironman is not your best first choice). Having a yearlong training approach gives you room to recover from any potential mishap, injury, or illness (hopefully minor ones). It also takes some pressure off by giving you plenty of time to gradually work your way to a higher level of fitness.

Ironman races generally fill up quickly, so it's important that you register early. Many championship-level races at this distance, such as the famous Ironman World Championship in Kona, Hawaii, may not even allow amateur competition or may allocate only a few lottery entries for the masses. If you are a competitive age-grouper, check to see which races in your area help you qualify for a championship-level Ironman race.

Costs can be a significant factor in your decision to race an Ironman, especially if the race of your choosing is a flight or two away. Besides the entry cost, you have to figure in airfare and lodging for multiple days. Always give yourself a few days for recovery after your Ironman triathlon, or you'll have a painfully long flight home.

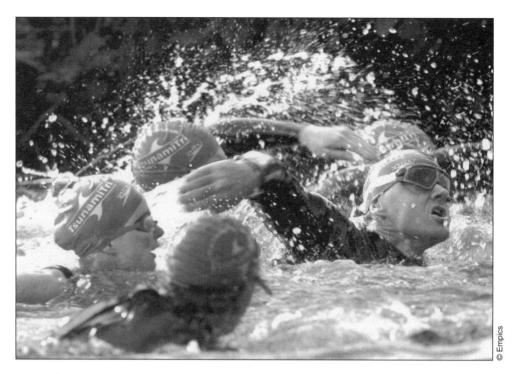

Ironman competition can be fierce. Make sure you go into the race with a sufficient level of preparation.

Ironman training demands a commitment of anywhere from 20 hours a week at a minimum to 30 or more hours weekly. As I've already hinted, this huge time commitment should not be entered into lightly.

As with all the workouts in this book, the Ironman workouts shown here are meant to give you a snapshot of what training might take for this event. It's particularly important to make sure that you build a good solid base of training before attempting some of the more demanding workouts shown in table 11.1.

To individualize your Ironman distance training, take into account the following factors:

- Current fitness level
- Goals
- Strengths
- Weaknesses
- Technical weaknesses (such as poor swimming technique)
- Injuries or other limitations
- Special disabilities
- Topography of race course
- Any other conditions of the race course

The sample workouts include a variety of approaches to working out: key workouts, heart rate training, and 80/20 workouts. Determine your most effective approach or use a variety to achieve your goals. Both time-based workouts and distance-based training are shown on the workout charts—use whichever you feel most comfortable with. You may find—particularly with the longer runs—that a training approach based on time can help you manage your time more efficiently, with less pressure to run a certain distance.

Like all the training grids, these usually give you Mondays off or recommend a recovery workout. For most of your Ironman training, you'll be doing some awfully tough work on weekends. That means your body and mind need those easy or off Mondays to recover.

Because of the demanding nature of Ironman training, it's especially important to back off on both the intensity and volume of your workouts in the two weeks before your race. You may be addicted to the high of long-distance training, but you owe it to yourself to be recovered and fresh on race day.

Customize your tapering to suit your unique needs. Some considerations for determining your ideal tapering schedule are the following:

- Your age
- Your rate of recovery from a workout
- Your intensity and volume of training in the month before the race
- Your travel time to a distant race
- Your mental state (if you're burned out on training, maybe you need a little more tapering)

With an Ironman distance event, you should consider a two-week tapering schedule. The list to the right recommends a total amount of time you should spend training. Simply divide the disciplines into the same proportions you've been doing or, if you'd like a little more recovery, focus on swimming drills and easy bike and runs.

Two-Week Ironman Taper

Day	
Day 1	90 min
Day 2	Complete rest
Day 3	60 min
Day 4	45 min
Day 5	45 min
Day 6	Complete rest
Day 7	60 min
Day 8	45 min
Day 9	Complete rest
Day 10	30 min
Day 11	30 min
Day 12	20 min
Day 13	Complete rest
Day 14	Race day

Table 11.1 Training Snapshot for an Ironman-Distance Triathlon

	Monday	Tuesday	Wednesday
Week 1	(KEY): Brainwork workout on p. 72, distance modified to 3800 m	(HR): 40 mi (64K) in recovery and endurance zone	: 45 min easy
Week 2	Recovery day (off)	(KEY): Race simulation workout on p. 73, distance modified to 3800 m	(HR): 50 mi (80K) in recovery and endurance zone
Week 3	Recovery day (off)	(KEY): Technique golf workout on p. 73, distance modified to 10 x 50 m	: 60 mi (97K) easy spinning at 90 RPM or higher
Week 4	Recovery day (off)	(KEY): Sustainable pace workout on p. 73	: 60 mi (97K) at moderate pace on a course that has a few challenging hills
Week 5	Recovery day (off)	(80/20): Race simulation swim in supervised open water for 70 min; or 60 min swim in pool, practicing navigational sighting skills	: 60 mi (97K) at a moderate pace
Week 6	Recovery day (off)	(KEY): Hold a pace workout on p. 74, distance modified to 10 x 100 m	: 50 mi (80K) at a moderate pace with 6 x 2 mi (3.2K) race pace efforts in the middle, 5 min recovery between efforts
Week 7	Recovery day (off) (or) : 1500 m easy followed by drill sets	(KEY): Countdown workout on p. 74, distance modified to a total of 3800 m by swimming a 900 m, 800 m, 600 m, 500 m, 400 m, 300 m, 200 m, 100 m	: Group ride of 50-60 mi (80-97K)
Week 8	Recovery day (off)	(KEY): Hard-easy-hard workout on p. 74, distance modified to 4 x 125 m fast speed, 2 x 125 m very easy, and 4 x 125 m fast speed	(interval): 1 mi (1.6K) easy warm-up; 3 x .25 mi, 2 x .50 mi; 1 x 1 mi, 2 x .25 mi, resting 1 min between intervals; 1 mi (1.6K) easy cool-down

Note: Although it is not always specified here, always warm up and cool down properly with an easy effort. When distance or time isn't specified, use your own discretion for completing the workout in a distance that's right for your current fitness and ability levels. Always create your own plan based on your current training stage and individual goals.

Thursday	Friday	Saturday	Sunday
(swim): 2000 m easy (bike): 90 min spinning at 90 RPM or higher	(swim): 1500 m followed by drills	(bike): 60 mi (97K) easy spinning at 90 RPM or higher	(run): 90 min easy
(run): 1 hr easy (swim): Drills	(swim) (KEY): Sustainable pace workout on p. 73	(bike): 75 mi (121K) easy spinning at 90 RPM or higher	(run) (HR): 90 min in recovery and endurance base zone (swim): Drills
(run): 1 hr run with 15 min at tempo pace in the middle portion (swim): 15 min easy warm-up followed by drill sets	(swim): 2200 m easy followed by drills	(bike) (HR): 75 mi (121K) in recovery and endurance zone	(run) (KEY): 90 min run—30 min easy, 30 min tempo run, 30 min easy
(run): 1 hr easy run	(swim): 1800 m followed by drill sets	(bike) (HR): 75 mi (121K) in recovery and endurance zone (swim): 15 min warm-up set followed by drill sets	(run) (HR): 90 min easy run in recovery and endurance zone
(run) (KEY): 45 min tempo run or HR run in aerobic and tempo zone	(swim): 2500 m easy, followed by drills	(bike) (KEY): 100 mi (161K) on a hilly course hill workout on p.79 for integrating a challenging HR workout with hills)	(run) (HR): 90 min easy run in recovery and endurance zone
(run): Group run of 8-10 mi (13-16K) at conversational pace, or 1 hr easy run	(swim) (KEY): Hard-easy-hard workout on p. 74, distance modified to 4 x 100 m fast speed, 2 x 100 m very easy, and 4 x 100 m fast speed	(bike): 25 mi (40K) easy spinning at 90 RPM or higher (or) (swim): 30 min easy followed by drill sets	(bike) / (run) brick (80/20) (bike): 75 mi (121K) at a moderate pace or in the aerobic and tempo zone (run): 70 min easy
(run): 40 min easy followed by 15 min at near race pace, 10 min easy cool-down	(swim) (KEY): Sustainable pace workout on p. 73, 2 x 1900 m (do not modify distance)	(bike) (HR): 40 mi (64K) in aerobic and tempo zone	(run) (HR): 18-20 mi (29-32K) in recovery and endurance base zone
(swim): 2400 m easy followed by drill sets	(run): 45 min easy	(bike) (HR): 60 mi (97K) in aerobic and tempo zone	(run): 14-16 mi (23-26K) in aerobic and tempo zone

CHAPTER 12

Logs and Workout Tracking Tools

When I look back at some of my first training logs, my initial reaction is to either choke away a tear or let go a hearty chuckle. I flip through the pages of my first running log and read a heartbreaking account of having to walk the last 10 miles of my first marathon because of a knee injury. I remember how hard I trained for that event, only to have my knee blow out on mile 16, and how distraught I was afterward.

Then I flip through my first triathlon log book and laugh quietly when I relive the zigzag route I took on my first triathlon open-water swim and the minor spill I had on the bike course. You'd think either of these events would have prompted me to throw in the towel. However, both motivated me to try all that much harder in the next race.

Whether your triathlon log causes you to sniffle or to snicker, there are many more reasons to document your training than a trip down memory lane. A good deal of the value of keeping training records is to remind you of past accomplishments. But keeping a record of your triathlon training and racing has more practical applications as well. By recording all your workouts in a log, you'll circumvent possible injury and improve your performance.

If you're feeling run-down and are experiencing mild joint pain, a quick review of your training logs can easily tell you whether you've had too many high-intensity or high-volume workouts strung too close together. Documentation of the cold, hard facts has a way of bringing reality to the forefront, and that's exactly what a training log is intended to do. Conversely, if you experience a great performance, reviewing your training in the months before the race and your tapering in the week or two preceding the event will give you gems of information that you can use for future personal best times.

Maintaining an accurate log of your daily and weekly swimming, biking, and running workouts is thus one of the best ways to keep on track. A diary that chronicles the variables that affect your energy level and performance can help you achieve your triathlon goals. Using the same methodology, you can also track the variables, training methods, and factors that lead to your best performances.

This chapter provides both the materials you need to create and maintain a successful training log and the planning resources you need to have a smile on your face at the finish line.

From setting your short- and long-term goals to planting milestones to planning your training week by week, the following tools will help ensure that you lay the groundwork for an effective, efficient, and safe triathlon season. The log pages include everything you need to document your workouts, including sections that specifically address the key workout method and the 80/20 workouts mentioned in previous chapters. Of course, it's always fun to take a look back and impress your friends with the astounding number of miles or kilometers you've accumulated in total training, so there's a summary tool to help you do just that.

Your triathlon goal planner (page 130) is a helpful planning tool to keep you on target through your training season, as described in chapter 1. Here's where you commit to your long-term race goals and pen some short-term goals that will help you get there efficiently with the performance that you seek. Once you've completed your plan, refer to the table often to make sure you are checking off the short-term goals. Don't hesitate to add other short-term goals that you feel will help you to the finish line during your training season; remember that training is an adaptive process, and you may learn new things or have training opportunities that you didn't originally anticipate. Last of all, this table will help motivate you as you cross off your completed short-term goals, recognizing that you are drawing ever closer to your ultimate target.

Your benchmark planner (page 131) will help you set personal benchmarks within your training season schedule (refer to chapter 3 if you need a refresher on setting benchmarks). Remember that benchmarks are progressive measuring sticks to help you determine that you are on track. Whether they are training races, organized bike rides, or local running events, these targets should build on each other and provide ever-increasing challenges. This table is a reality check—a valuable tool to ensure that you have no delusions about your training progress.

The eight-week training log at the end of this chapter is comprised of three types of forms, each designed to help you plan and track your training on a daily, weekly, or monthly basis. Use the weekly planning worksheet to plan your training for the week. It's important to take some time on a Sunday evening or some time before the beginning of a training week to sit back, reflect on goals for the coming week, and plan your training appropriately. Getting into this habit will motivate you as you look forward to the week of training ahead and make any appropriate changes in your schedule. Again, be smart and adaptive and adjust your weekly training schedule as needed. Planning on a weekly basis also helps you balance

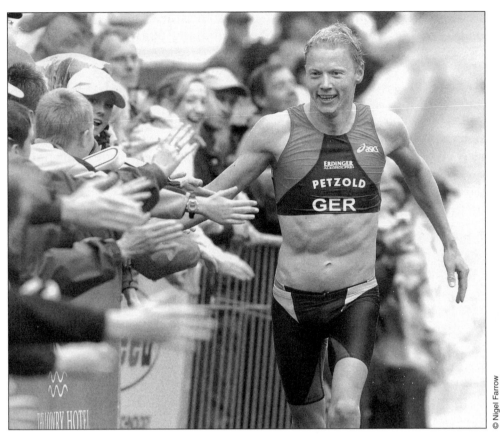

There is no greater feeling than reveling in the applause of race spectators at the finish line. Planning effective workouts is your first step in getting there.

© Nigel Farrow

your priorities—be diligent about making sure that the other important aspects of your life do not suffer when you look at the next seven days.

Use the daily training log pages to keep track of your daily workouts. Although you may not need or want to complete all the information, the more detailed your records, the better the value and functionality of your training log. Remember—in order to nail down the variables that can contribute to your greatest performance or the clues that can help you avoid injury, you'll need to be diligent and detailed about your training records. Commit to a specific time to complete your log. The best time to do so is immediately after a workout, when your mind is fresh and your spirit is roused by the high of exercise.

Use the monthly training summary page, located at the end of the eight-week training log, to track your year-to-date (or training season) totals, as well as your monthly sums. If you prefer to train using time-based measurements, you can use these pages to track minutes or a combination of distance and time. Finally, several blank notes pages are provided at the end of this chapter.

Triathlon is a wonderful sport that combines three heart-pounding disciplines into one exhilarating, adrenaline-pumping, empowering experience. Designing, creating, and capturing that experience takes forethought and planning. As with anything good you want to happen in your life, you've got to attend to it on a regular basis, with intelligence and a bit of artistic improvisation.

It's my wish that the planning tools and log pages in this book give you the valuable resources you need to reach your triathlon goals, while also giving you the flexibility to adapt your training to suit your unique needs.

Dream. Plan. Do. And most of all—enjoy!

Table 12.1   Your Goal Planner

Long-term goal	Deadline or metric
Short-term goals	**Race date:**

Table 12.2 Your Benchmark Planner

Benchmark description	How will this help you achieve your long-term goal? Why is it important?	Target date

Weekly Planning Worksheet

This week's goal: _____

Training stage (circle one):   Base   STS   Peak   Tapering

	Workout activity	Distance or time	Type or intensity	Course	Notes
Monday					
Tuesday					
Wednesday					
Thursday					
Friday					
Saturday					
Sunday					

Target distance or time totals for this week:

Swim: _____   Bike: _____   Run: _____

Daily Training Log

Today's Goal

Days until race: _____

Today's Stats

Today's date:_____   Conditions:_____

Time of day: _____   Course: _____

Temperature:_____   Training partners: _____

80/20 Workout

☐ Intervals   ☐ Brick   ☐ Race simulation   ☐ Weakness   ☐ Power

Is this also a key workout?   ☐ Yes   ☐ No

Importance of 80/20 rule to goal: ☐ High   ☐ Moderate   ☐ Low

Workout Information

Discipline:	☐ Swim	☐ Bike	☐ Run	☐ Other
Distances:	_____	_____	_____	_____
Total time:	_____	_____	_____	_____
Intensity:	_____	_____	_____	_____

Other Details

Warm-up: _____   Cool-down: _____   Flexibility training: _____

Strength training: Weights _____   Sets _____   Reps _____

Results and Observations

Pace: _____   Splits: _____

Heart rate training: Resting heart rate: _____

Target zone: ☐ Recovery/endurance   ☐ Aerobic/tempo   ☐ Anaerobic threshold

% time spent in target zone: _____

Injury or overtraining flags: Joint soreness   ☐ Yes   ☐ No

Moodiness   ☐ Yes   ☐ No

Slow recovery   ☐ Yes   ☐ No

Other: _____

Training and Nutrition Notes

Daily Training Log

Today's Goal   *Days until race:* _____

Today's Stats

Today's date:_____   Conditions:_____

Time of day: _____   Course: _____

Temperature:_____   Training partners: _____

80/20 Workout

☐ Intervals   ☐ Brick   ☐ Race simulation   ☐ Weakness   ☐ Power

Is this also a key workout?   ☐ Yes   ☐ No

Importance of 80/20 rule to goal: ☐ High   ☐ Moderate   ☐ Low

Workout Information

Discipline:	☐ Swim	☐ Bike	☐ Run	☐ Other
Distances:	_____	_____	_____	_____
Total time:	_____	_____	_____	_____
Intensity:	_____	_____	_____	_____

Other Details

Warm-up: _____   Cool-down: _____   Flexibility training: _____

Strength training: Weights _____   Sets _____   Reps _____

Results and Observations

Pace: _____   Splits: _____

Heart rate training: Resting heart rate: _____

Target zone: ☐ Recovery/endurance   ☐ Aerobic/tempo   ☐ Anaerobic threshold

% time spent in target zone: _____

Injury or overtraining flags: Joint soreness   ☐ Yes   ☐ No

Moodiness   ☐ Yes   ☐ No

Slow recovery   ☐ Yes   ☐ No

Other: _____

Training and Nutrition Notes

Daily Training Log

Today's Goal

Days until race: _____

Today's Stats

Today's date: _____   Conditions: _____

Time of day: _____   Course: _____

Temperature: _____   Training partners: _____

80/20 Workout

☐ Intervals   ☐ Brick   ☐ Race simulation   ☐ Weakness   ☐ Power

Is this also a key workout?   ☐ Yes   ☐ No

Importance of 80/20 rule to goal: ☐ High   ☐ Moderate   ☐ Low

Workout Information

Discipline:	☐ Swim	☐ Bike	☐ Run	☐ Other
Distances:	_____	_____	_____	_____
Total time:	_____	_____	_____	_____
Intensity:	_____	_____	_____	_____

Other Details

Warm-up: _____   Cool-down: _____   Flexibility training: _____

Strength training: Weights _____   Sets _____   Reps _____

Results and Observations

Pace: _____   Splits: _____

Heart rate training: Resting heart rate: _____

Target zone: ☐ Recovery/endurance   ☐ Aerobic/tempo   ☐ Anaerobic threshold

% time spent in target zone: _____

Injury or overtraining flags:	Joint soreness	☐ Yes	☐ No
	Moodiness	☐ Yes	☐ No
	Slow recovery	☐ Yes	☐ No
	Other: _____		

Training and Nutrition Notes

Daily Training Log

Today's Goal

Days until race: _____

Today's Stats

Today's date: _____   Conditions: _____

Time of day: _____   Course: _____

Temperature: _____   Training partners: _____

80/20 Workout

☐ Intervals   ☐ Brick   ☐ Race simulation   ☐ Weakness   ☐ Power

Is this also a key workout?   ☐ Yes   ☐ No

Importance of 80/20 rule to goal: ☐ High   ☐ Moderate   ☐ Low

Workout Information

Discipline: ☐ Swim   ☐ Bike   ☐ Run   ☐ Other

Distances: _____   _____   _____   _____

Total time: _____   _____   _____   _____

Intensity: _____   _____   _____   _____

Other Details

Warm-up: _____   Cool-down: _____   Flexibility training: _____

Strength training: Weights _____   Sets _____   Reps _____

Results and Observations

Pace: _____   Splits: _____

Heart rate training: Resting heart rate: _____

Target zone: ☐ Recovery/endurance   ☐ Aerobic/tempo   ☐ Anaerobic threshold

% time spent in target zone: _____

Injury or overtraining flags: Joint soreness   ☐ Yes   ☐ No

                                                    Moodiness   ☐ Yes   ☐ No

                                                    Slow recovery   ☐ Yes   ☐ No

                                                    Other: _____

Training and Nutrition Notes

Daily Training Log

Today's Goal   **Days until race:** _____

Today's Stats

Today's date: _____   Conditions: _____

Time of day: _____   Course: _____

Temperature: _____   Training partners: _____

80/20 Workout

☐ Intervals   ☐ Brick   ☐ Race simulation   ☐ Weakness   ☐ Power

Is this also a key workout?   ☐ Yes   ☐ No

Importance of 80/20 rule to goal: ☐ High   ☐ Moderate   ☐ Low

Workout Information

Discipline: ☐ Swim   ☐ Bike   ☐ Run   ☐ Other

Distances: _____   _____   _____   _____

Total time: _____   _____   _____   _____

Intensity: _____   _____   _____   _____

Other Details

Warm-up: _____   Cool-down: _____   Flexibility training: _____

Strength training: Weights _____   Sets _____   Reps _____

Results and Observations

Pace: _____   Splits: _____

Heart rate training: Resting heart rate: _____

Target zone: ☐ Recovery/endurance   ☐ Aerobic/tempo   ☐ Anaerobic threshold

% time spent in target zone: _____

Injury or overtraining flags: Joint soreness   ☐ Yes   ☐ No

                                         Moodiness   ☐ Yes   ☐ No

                                         Slow recovery   ☐ Yes   ☐ No

                                         Other: _____

Training and Nutrition Notes

Daily Training Log

Today's Goal   *Days until race:* _____

Today's Stats

Today's date: _____   Conditions: _____

Time of day: _____   Course: _____

Temperature: _____   Training partners: _____

80/20 Workout

☐ Intervals   ☐ Brick   ☐ Race simulation   ☐ Weakness   ☐ Power

Is this also a key workout?   ☐ Yes   ☐ No

Importance of 80/20 rule to goal: ☐ High   ☐ Moderate   ☐ Low

Workout Information

Discipline: ☐ Swim   ☐ Bike   ☐ Run   ☐ Other

Distances: _____   _____   _____   _____

Total time: _____   _____   _____   _____

Intensity: _____   _____   _____   _____

Other Details

Warm-up: _____   Cool-down: _____   Flexibility training: _____

Strength training: Weights _____   Sets _____   Reps _____

Results and Observations

Pace: _____   Splits: _____

Heart rate training: Resting heart rate: _____

Target zone: ☐ Recovery/endurance   ☐ Aerobic/tempo   ☐ Anaerobic threshold

% time spent in target zone: _____

Injury or overtraining flags: Joint soreness   ☐ Yes   ☐ No

                                                           Moodiness   ☐ Yes   ☐ No

                                                           Slow recovery   ☐ Yes   ☐ No

                                                           Other: _____

Training and Nutrition Notes

Daily Training Log

Today's Goal   *Days until race:* _____

Today's Stats

Today's date: _____   Conditions: _____

Time of day: _____   Course: _____

Temperature: _____   Training partners: _____

80/20 Workout

☐ Intervals   ☐ Brick   ☐ Race simulation   ☐ Weakness   ☐ Power

Is this also a key workout?   ☐ Yes   ☐ No

Importance of 80/20 rule to goal: ☐ High   ☐ Moderate   ☐ Low

Workout Information

Discipline: ☐ Swim   ☐ Bike   ☐ Run   ☐ Other

Distances: _____   _____   _____   _____

Total time: _____   _____   _____   _____

Intensity: _____   _____   _____   _____

Other Details

Warm-up: _____   Cool-down: _____   Flexibility training: _____

Strength training: Weights _____   Sets _____   Reps _____

Results and Observations

Pace: _____   Splits: _____

Heart rate training: Resting heart rate: _____

Target zone: ☐ Recovery/endurance   ☐ Aerobic/tempo   ☐ Anaerobic threshold

% time spent in target zone: _____

Injury or overtraining flags: Joint soreness   ☐ Yes   ☐ No

                                          Moodiness   ☐ Yes   ☐ No

                                          Slow recovery   ☐ Yes   ☐ No

                                          Other: _____

Training and Nutrition Notes

Weekly Planning Worksheet

This week's goal: _____

Training stage (circle one):   Base   STS   Peak   Tapering

	Workout activity	Distance or time	Type or intensity	Course	Notes
Monday					
Tuesday					
Wednesday					
Thursday					
Friday					
Saturday					
Sunday					

Target distance or time totals for this week:

Swim: _____   Bike: _____   Run: _____

Daily Training Log

Today's Goal   ***Days until race:*** _____

Today's Stats

Today's date: _____   Conditions: _____

Time of day: _____   Course: _____

Temperature: _____   Training partners: _____

80/20 Workout

☐ Intervals   ☐ Brick   ☐ Race simulation   ☐ Weakness   ☐ Power

Is this also a key workout?   ☐ Yes   ☐ No

Importance of 80/20 rule to goal: ☐ High   ☐ Moderate   ☐ Low

Workout Information

Discipline:	☐ Swim	☐ Bike	☐ Run	☐ Other
Distances:	_____	_____	_____	_____
Total time:	_____	_____	_____	_____
Intensity:	_____	_____	_____	_____

Other Details

Warm-up: _____   Cool-down: _____   Flexibility training: _____

Strength training: Weights _____   Sets _____   Reps _____

Results and Observations

Pace: _____   Splits: _____

Heart rate training: Resting heart rate: _____

Target zone: ☐ Recovery/endurance   ☐ Aerobic/tempo   ☐ Anaerobic threshold

% time spent in target zone: _____

Injury or overtraining flags: Joint soreness   ☐ Yes   ☐ No

Moodiness   ☐ Yes   ☐ No

Slow recovery   ☐ Yes   ☐ No

Other: _____

Training and Nutrition Notes

Daily Training Log

Today's Goal   *Days until race:* _____

Today's Stats

Today's date:_____   Conditions:_____

Time of day: _____   Course: _____

Temperature:_____   Training partners: _____

80/20 Workout

☐ Intervals   ☐ Brick   ☐ Race simulation   ☐ Weakness   ☐ Power

Is this also a key workout?   ☐ Yes   ☐ No

Importance of 80/20 rule to goal: ☐ High   ☐ Moderate   ☐ Low

Workout Information

Discipline: ☐ Swim   ☐ Bike   ☐ Run   ☐ Other

Distances: _____   _____   _____   _____

Total time: _____   _____   _____   _____

Intensity: _____   _____   _____   _____

Other Details

Warm-up: _____   Cool-down: _____   Flexibility training: _____

Strength training: Weights _____   Sets _____   Reps _____

Results and Observations

Pace: _____   Splits: _____

Heart rate training: Resting heart rate: _____

Target zone: ☐ Recovery/endurance   ☐ Aerobic/tempo   ☐ Anaerobic threshold

% time spent in target zone: _____

Injury or overtraining flags: Joint soreness   ☐ Yes   ☐ No

                                   Moodiness   ☐ Yes   ☐ No

                                   Slow recovery   ☐ Yes   ☐ No

                                   Other: _____

Training and Nutrition Notes

Daily Training Log

Today's Goal

Days until race: _____

Today's Stats

Today's date: _____   Conditions: _____

Time of day: _____   Course: _____

Temperature: _____   Training partners: _____

80/20 Workout

☐ Intervals   ☐ Brick   ☐ Race simulation   ☐ Weakness   ☐ Power

Is this also a key workout?   ☐ Yes   ☐ No

Importance of 80/20 rule to goal: ☐ High   ☐ Moderate   ☐ Low

Workout Information

Discipline: ☐ Swim   ☐ Bike   ☐ Run   ☐ Other

Distances: _____   _____   _____   _____

Total time: _____   _____   _____   _____

Intensity: _____   _____   _____   _____

Other Details

Warm-up: _____   Cool-down: _____   Flexibility training: _____

Strength training: Weights _____   Sets _____   Reps _____

Results and Observations

Pace: _____   Splits: _____

Heart rate training: Resting heart rate: _____

Target zone: ☐ Recovery/endurance   ☐ Aerobic/tempo   ☐ Anaerobic threshold

% time spent in target zone: _____

Injury or overtraining flags: Joint soreness   ☐ Yes   ☐ No

Moodiness   ☐ Yes   ☐ No

Slow recovery   ☐ Yes   ☐ No

Other: _____

Training and Nutrition Notes

Daily Training Log

Today's Goal   ***Days until race:*** _____

Today's Stats

Today's date:_____   Conditions:_____

Time of day: _____   Course: _____

Temperature:_____   Training partners: _____

80/20 Workout

☐ Intervals   ☐ Brick   ☐ Race simulation   ☐ Weakness   ☐ Power

Is this also a key workout?   ☐ Yes   ☐ No

Importance of 80/20 rule to goal: ☐ High   ☐ Moderate   ☐ Low

Workout Information

Discipline: ☐ Swim   ☐ Bike   ☐ Run   ☐ Other

Distances: _____   _____   _____   _____

Total time: _____   _____   _____   _____

Intensity: _____   _____   _____   _____

Other Details

Warm-up: _____   Cool-down: _____   Flexibility training: _____

Strength training: Weights _____   Sets _____   Reps _____

Results and Observations

Pace: _____   Splits: _____

Heart rate training: Resting heart rate: _____

Target zone: ☐ Recovery/endurance   ☐ Aerobic/tempo   ☐ Anaerobic threshold

% time spent in target zone: _____

Injury or overtraining flags: Joint soreness   ☐ Yes   ☐ No

                                                          Moodiness   ☐ Yes   ☐ No

                                                          Slow recovery   ☐ Yes   ☐ No

                                                          Other: _____

Training and Nutrition Notes

Daily Training Log

Today's Goal

Days until race: _____

Today's Stats

Today's date: _____   Conditions: _____

Time of day: _____   Course: _____

Temperature: _____   Training partners: _____

80/20 Workout

☐ Intervals   ☐ Brick   ☐ Race simulation   ☐ Weakness   ☐ Power

Is this also a key workout?   ☐ Yes   ☐ No

Importance of 80/20 rule to goal: ☐ High   ☐ Moderate   ☐ Low

Workout Information

Discipline:	☐ Swim	☐ Bike	☐ Run	☐ Other
Distances:	_____	_____	_____	_____
Total time:	_____	_____	_____	_____
Intensity:	_____	_____	_____	_____

Other Details

Warm-up: _____   Cool-down: _____   Flexibility training: _____

Strength training: Weights _____   Sets _____   Reps _____

Results and Observations

Pace: _____   Splits: _____

Heart rate training: Resting heart rate: _____

Target zone: ☐ Recovery/endurance   ☐ Aerobic/tempo   ☐ Anaerobic threshold

% time spent in target zone: _____

Injury or overtraining flags: Joint soreness   ☐ Yes   ☐ No

Moodiness   ☐ Yes   ☐ No

Slow recovery   ☐ Yes   ☐ No

Other: _____

Training and Nutrition Notes

Daily Training Log

Today's Goal

Days until race: _____

Today's Stats

Today's date: _____   Conditions: _____

Time of day: _____   Course: _____

Temperature: _____   Training partners: _____

80/20 Workout

☐ Intervals   ☐ Brick   ☐ Race simulation   ☐ Weakness   ☐ Power

Is this also a key workout?   ☐ Yes   ☐ No

Importance of 80/20 rule to goal: ☐ High   ☐ Moderate   ☐ Low

Workout Information

Discipline:	☐ Swim	☐ Bike	☐ Run	☐ Other
Distances:	_____	_____	_____	_____
Total time:	_____	_____	_____	_____
Intensity:	_____	_____	_____	_____

Other Details

Warm-up: _____   Cool-down: _____   Flexibility training: _____

Strength training: Weights _____   Sets _____   Reps _____

Results and Observations

Pace: _____   Splits: _____

Heart rate training: Resting heart rate: _____

Target zone: ☐ Recovery/endurance   ☐ Aerobic/tempo   ☐ Anaerobic threshold

% time spent in target zone: _____

Injury or overtraining flags:	Joint soreness	☐ Yes	☐ No
	Moodiness	☐ Yes	☐ No
	Slow recovery	☐ Yes	☐ No
	Other: _____		

Training and Nutrition Notes

Daily Training Log

Today's Goal

Days until race: _____

Today's Stats

Today's date: _____   Conditions: _____

Time of day: _____   Course: _____

Temperature: _____   Training partners: _____

80/20 Workout

☐ Intervals   ☐ Brick   ☐ Race simulation   ☐ Weakness   ☐ Power

Is this also a key workout?   ☐ Yes   ☐ No

Importance of 80/20 rule to goal: ☐ High   ☐ Moderate   ☐ Low

Workout Information

Discipline:	☐ Swim	☐ Bike	☐ Run	☐ Other
Distances:	_____	_____	_____	_____
Total time:	_____	_____	_____	_____
Intensity:	_____	_____	_____	_____

Other Details

Warm-up: _____   Cool-down: _____   Flexibility training: _____

Strength training: Weights _____   Sets _____   Reps _____

Results and Observations

Pace: _____   Splits: _____

Heart rate training: Resting heart rate: _____

Target zone: ☐ Recovery/endurance   ☐ Aerobic/tempo   ☐ Anaerobic threshold

% time spent in target zone: _____

Injury or overtraining flags: Joint soreness   ☐ Yes   ☐ No

Moodiness   ☐ Yes   ☐ No

Slow recovery   ☐ Yes   ☐ No

Other: _____

Training and Nutrition Notes

Weekly Planning Worksheet

This week's goal: _____

Training stage (circle one):   Base   STS   Peak   Tapering

	Workout activity	Distance or time	Type or intensity	Course	Notes
Monday					
Tuesday					
Wednesday					
Thursday					
Friday					
Saturday					
Sunday					

Target distance or time totals for this week:

Swim: _____   Bike: _____   Run: _____

Daily Training Log

Today's Goal   *Days until race:* _____

Today's Stats

Today's date:_____   Conditions:_____

Time of day: _____   Course: _____

Temperature:_____   Training partners: _____

80/20 Workout

☐ Intervals   ☐ Brick   ☐ Race simulation   ☐ Weakness   ☐ Power

Is this also a key workout?   ☐ Yes   ☐ No

Importance of 80/20 rule to goal: ☐ High   ☐ Moderate   ☐ Low

Workout Information

Discipline: ☐ Swim   ☐ Bike   ☐ Run   ☐ Other

Distances: _____   _____   _____   _____

Total time: _____   _____   _____   _____

Intensity: _____   _____   _____   _____

Other Details

Warm-up: _____   Cool-down: _____   Flexibility training: _____

Strength training: Weights _____   Sets _____   Reps _____

Results and Observations

Pace: _____   Splits: _____

Heart rate training: Resting heart rate: _____

Target zone: ☐ Recovery/endurance   ☐ Aerobic/tempo   ☐ Anaerobic threshold

% time spent in target zone: _____

Injury or overtraining flags: Joint soreness   ☐ Yes   ☐ No

                                                     Moodiness   ☐ Yes   ☐ No

                                                     Slow recovery   ☐ Yes   ☐ No

                                                     Other: _____

Training and Nutrition Notes

Daily Training Log

Today's Goal   **Days until race:** _____

Today's Stats

Today's date: _____   Conditions: _____

Time of day: _____   Course: _____

Temperature: _____   Training partners: _____

80/20 Workout

☐ Intervals   ☐ Brick   ☐ Race simulation   ☐ Weakness   ☐ Power

Is this also a key workout?   ☐ Yes   ☐ No

Importance of 80/20 rule to goal: ☐ High   ☐ Moderate   ☐ Low

Workout Information

Discipline: ☐ Swim   ☐ Bike   ☐ Run   ☐ Other

Distances: _____   _____   _____   _____

Total time: _____   _____   _____   _____

Intensity: _____   _____   _____   _____

Other Details

Warm-up: _____   Cool-down: _____   Flexibility training: _____

Strength training: Weights _____   Sets _____   Reps _____

Results and Observations

Pace: _____   Splits: _____

Heart rate training: Resting heart rate: _____

Target zone: ☐ Recovery/endurance   ☐ Aerobic/tempo   ☐ Anaerobic threshold

% time spent in target zone: _____

Injury or overtraining flags: Joint soreness   ☐ Yes   ☐ No

Moodiness   ☐ Yes   ☐ No

Slow recovery   ☐ Yes   ☐ No

Other: _____

Training and Nutrition Notes

Daily Training Log

Today's Goal   *Days until race:* _____

Today's Stats

Today's date: _____   Conditions: _____

Time of day: _____   Course: _____

Temperature: _____   Training partners: _____

80/20 Workout

☐ Intervals   ☐ Brick   ☐ Race simulation   ☐ Weakness   ☐ Power

Is this also a key workout?   ☐ Yes   ☐ No

Importance of 80/20 rule to goal: ☐ High   ☐ Moderate   ☐ Low

Workout Information

Discipline: ☐ Swim   ☐ Bike   ☐ Run   ☐ Other

Distances: _____   _____   _____   _____

Total time: _____   _____   _____   _____

Intensity: _____   _____   _____   _____

Other Details

Warm-up: _____   Cool-down: _____   Flexibility training: _____

Strength training: Weights _____   Sets _____   Reps _____

Results and Observations

Pace: _____   Splits: _____

Heart rate training: Resting heart rate: _____

Target zone: ☐ Recovery/endurance   ☐ Aerobic/tempo   ☐ Anaerobic threshold

% time spent in target zone: _____

Injury or overtraining flags: Joint soreness   ☐ Yes   ☐ No

                                      Moodiness   ☐ Yes   ☐ No

                                      Slow recovery   ☐ Yes   ☐ No

                                      Other: _____

Training and Nutrition Notes

Daily Training Log

Today's Goal

Days until race: _____

Today's Stats

Today's date:_____   Conditions:_____

Time of day: _____   Course: _____

Temperature:_____   Training partners: _____

80/20 Workout

☐ Intervals   ☐ Brick   ☐ Race simulation   ☐ Weakness   ☐ Power

Is this also a key workout?   ☐ Yes   ☐ No

Importance of 80/20 rule to goal: ☐ High   ☐ Moderate   ☐ Low

Workout Information

Discipline:	☐ Swim	☐ Bike	☐ Run	☐ Other
Distances:	_____	_____	_____	_____
Total time:	_____	_____	_____	_____
Intensity:	_____	_____	_____	_____

Other Details

Warm-up: _____   Cool-down: _____   Flexibility training: _____

Strength training: Weights _____   Sets _____   Reps _____

Results and Observations

Pace: _____   Splits: _____

Heart rate training: Resting heart rate: _____

Target zone: ☐ Recovery/endurance   ☐ Aerobic/tempo   ☐ Anaerobic threshold

% time spent in target zone: _____

Injury or overtraining flags:

Joint soreness   ☐ Yes   ☐ No

Moodiness   ☐ Yes   ☐ No

Slow recovery   ☐ Yes   ☐ No

Other: _____

Training and Nutrition Notes

Daily Training Log

Today's Goal

Days until race: _____

Today's Stats

Today's date: _____   Conditions: _____

Time of day: _____   Course: _____

Temperature: _____   Training partners: _____

80/20 Workout

☐ Intervals   ☐ Brick   ☐ Race simulation   ☐ Weakness   ☐ Power

Is this also a key workout?   ☐ Yes   ☐ No

Importance of 80/20 rule to goal: ☐ High   ☐ Moderate   ☐ Low

Workout Information

Discipline:	☐ Swim	☐ Bike	☐ Run	☐ Other
Distances:	_____	_____	_____	_____
Total time:	_____	_____	_____	_____
Intensity:	_____	_____	_____	_____

Other Details

Warm-up: _____   Cool-down: _____   Flexibility training: _____

Strength training: Weights _____   Sets _____   Reps _____

Results and Observations

Pace: _____   Splits: _____

Heart rate training: Resting heart rate: _____

Target zone: ☐ Recovery/endurance   ☐ Aerobic/tempo   ☐ Anaerobic threshold

% time spent in target zone: _____

Injury or overtraining flags:	Joint soreness	☐ Yes	☐ No
	Moodiness	☐ Yes	☐ No
	Slow recovery	☐ Yes	☐ No
	Other: _____		

Training and Nutrition Notes

Daily Training Log

Today's Goal   ***Days until race:*** _____

Today's Stats

Today's date: _____   Conditions: _____

Time of day: _____   Course: _____

Temperature: _____   Training partners: _____

80/20 Workout

☐ Intervals   ☐ Brick   ☐ Race simulation   ☐ Weakness   ☐ Power

Is this also a key workout?   ☐ Yes   ☐ No

Importance of 80/20 rule to goal: ☐ High   ☐ Moderate   ☐ Low

Workout Information

Discipline:	☐ Swim	☐ Bike	☐ Run	☐ Other
Distances:	_____	_____	_____	_____
Total time:	_____	_____	_____	_____
Intensity:	_____	_____	_____	_____

Other Details

Warm-up: _____   Cool-down: _____   Flexibility training: _____

Strength training: Weights _____   Sets _____   Reps _____

Results and Observations

Pace: _____   Splits: _____

Heart rate training: Resting heart rate: _____

Target zone: ☐ Recovery/endurance   ☐ Aerobic/tempo   ☐ Anaerobic threshold

% time spent in target zone: _____

Injury or overtraining flags: Joint soreness   ☐ Yes   ☐ No

Moodiness   ☐ Yes   ☐ No

Slow recovery   ☐ Yes   ☐ No

Other: _____

Training and Nutrition Notes

Daily Training Log

Today's Goal   **Days until race:** _____

Today's Stats

Today's date:_____   Conditions:_____

Time of day: _____   Course: _____

Temperature:_____   Training partners: _____

80/20 Workout

☐ Intervals   ☐ Brick   ☐ Race simulation   ☐ Weakness   ☐ Power

Is this also a key workout?   ☐ Yes   ☐ No

Importance of 80/20 rule to goal: ☐ High   ☐ Moderate   ☐ Low

Workout Information

Discipline:	☐ Swim	☐ Bike	☐ Run	☐ Other
Distances:	_____	_____	_____	_____
Total time:	_____	_____	_____	_____
Intensity:	_____	_____	_____	_____

Other Details

Warm-up: _____   Cool-down: _____   Flexibility training: _____

Strength training: Weights _____   Sets _____   Reps _____

Results and Observations

Pace: _____   Splits: _____

Heart rate training: Resting heart rate: _____

Target zone: ☐ Recovery/endurance   ☐ Aerobic/tempo   ☐ Anaerobic threshold

% time spent in target zone: _____

Injury or overtraining flags: Joint soreness   ☐ Yes   ☐ No

Moodiness   ☐ Yes   ☐ No

Slow recovery   ☐ Yes   ☐ No

Other: _____

Training and Nutrition Notes

Weekly Planning Worksheet

This week's goal: _____

Training stage (circle one):   Base   STS   Peak   Tapering

	Workout activity	Distance or time	Type or intensity	Course	Notes
Monday					
Tuesday					
Wednesday					
Thursday					
Friday					
Saturday					
Sunday					

Target distance or time totals for this week:

Swim: _____   Bike: _____   Run: _____

Daily Training Log

Today's Goal   **Days until race:** _____

Today's Stats

Today's date: _____   Conditions: _____

Time of day: _____   Course: _____

Temperature: _____   Training partners: _____

80/20 Workout

□ Intervals   □ Brick   □ Race simulation   □ Weakness   □ Power

Is this also a key workout?   □ Yes   □ No

Importance of 80/20 rule to goal: □ High   □ Moderate   □ Low

Workout Information

Discipline:	□ Swim	□ Bike	□ Run	□ Other
Distances:	_____	_____	_____	_____
Total time:	_____	_____	_____	_____
Intensity:	_____	_____	_____	_____

Other Details

Warm-up: _____   Cool-down: _____   Flexibility training: _____

Strength training: Weights _____   Sets _____   Reps _____

Results and Observations

Pace: _____   Splits: _____

Heart rate training: Resting heart rate: _____

Target zone: □ Recovery/endurance   □ Aerobic/tempo   □ Anaerobic threshold

% time spent in target zone: _____

Injury or overtraining flags: Joint soreness   □ Yes   □ No

Moodiness   □ Yes   □ No

Slow recovery   □ Yes   □ No

Other: _____

Training and Nutrition Notes

Daily Training Log

Today's Goal

Days until race: _____

Today's Stats

Today's date:_____   Conditions:_____

Time of day: _____   Course: _____

Temperature:_____   Training partners: _____

80/20 Workout

☐ Intervals   ☐ Brick   ☐ Race simulation   ☐ Weakness   ☐ Power

Is this also a key workout?   ☐ Yes   ☐ No

Importance of 80/20 rule to goal: ☐ High   ☐ Moderate   ☐ Low

Workout Information

Discipline: ☐ Swim   ☐ Bike   ☐ Run   ☐ Other

Distances: _____   _____   _____   _____

Total time: _____   _____   _____   _____

Intensity: _____   _____   _____   _____

Other Details

Warm-up: _____   Cool-down: _____   Flexibility training: _____

Strength training: Weights _____   Sets _____   Reps _____

Results and Observations

Pace: _____   Splits: _____

Heart rate training: Resting heart rate: _____

Target zone: ☐ Recovery/endurance   ☐ Aerobic/tempo   ☐ Anaerobic threshold

% time spent in target zone: _____

Injury or overtraining flags: Joint soreness   ☐ Yes   ☐ No

Moodiness   ☐ Yes   ☐ No

Slow recovery   ☐ Yes   ☐ No

Other: _____

Training and Nutrition Notes

Daily Training Log

Today's Goal

Days until race: _____

Today's Stats

Today's date: _____   Conditions: _____

Time of day: _____   Course: _____

Temperature: _____   Training partners: _____

80/20 Workout

☐ Intervals   ☐ Brick   ☐ Race simulation   ☐ Weakness   ☐ Power

Is this also a key workout?   ☐ Yes   ☐ No

Importance of 80/20 rule to goal: ☐ High   ☐ Moderate   ☐ Low

Workout Information

Discipline:	☐ Swim	☐ Bike	☐ Run	☐ Other
Distances:	_____	_____	_____	_____
Total time:	_____	_____	_____	_____
Intensity:	_____	_____	_____	_____

Other Details

Warm-up: _____   Cool-down: _____   Flexibility training: _____

Strength training: Weights _____   Sets _____   Reps _____

Results and Observations

Pace: _____   Splits: _____

Heart rate training: Resting heart rate: _____

Target zone: ☐ Recovery/endurance   ☐ Aerobic/tempo   ☐ Anaerobic threshold

% time spent in target zone: _____

Injury or overtraining flags: Joint soreness   ☐ Yes   ☐ No

Moodiness   ☐ Yes   ☐ No

Slow recovery   ☐ Yes   ☐ No

Other: _____

Training and Nutrition Notes

Daily Training Log

Today's Goal

Days until race: _____

Today's Stats

Today's date: _____   Conditions: _____

Time of day: _____   Course: _____

Temperature: _____   Training partners: _____

80/20 Workout

☐ Intervals   ☐ Brick   ☐ Race simulation   ☐ Weakness   ☐ Power

Is this also a key workout?   ☐ Yes   ☐ No

Importance of 80/20 rule to goal: ☐ High   ☐ Moderate   ☐ Low

Workout Information

Discipline: ☐ Swim   ☐ Bike   ☐ Run   ☐ Other

Distances: _____   _____   _____   _____

Total time: _____   _____   _____   _____

Intensity: _____   _____   _____   _____

Other Details

Warm-up: _____   Cool-down: _____   Flexibility training: _____

Strength training: Weights _____   Sets _____   Reps _____

Results and Observations

Pace: _____   Splits: _____

Heart rate training: Resting heart rate: _____

Target zone: ☐ Recovery/endurance   ☐ Aerobic/tempo   ☐ Anaerobic threshold

% time spent in target zone: _____

Injury or overtraining flags: Joint soreness   ☐ Yes   ☐ No

Moodiness   ☐ Yes   ☐ No

Slow recovery   ☐ Yes   ☐ No

Other: _____

Training and Nutrition Notes

Daily Training Log

Today's Goal

Days until race: _____

Today's Stats

Today's date:_____   Conditions:_____

Time of day: _____   Course: _____

Temperature:_____   Training partners: _____

80/20 Workout

☐ Intervals   ☐ Brick   ☐ Race simulation   ☐ Weakness   ☐ Power

Is this also a key workout?   ☐ Yes   ☐ No

Importance of 80/20 rule to goal: ☐ High   ☐ Moderate   ☐ Low

Workout Information

Discipline: ☐ Swim   ☐ Bike   ☐ Run   ☐ Other

Distances: _____   _____   _____   _____

Total time: _____   _____   _____   _____

Intensity: _____   _____   _____   _____

Other Details

Warm-up: _____   Cool-down: _____   Flexibility training: _____

Strength training: Weights _____   Sets _____   Reps _____

Results and Observations

Pace: _____   Splits: _____

Heart rate training: Resting heart rate: _____

Target zone: ☐ Recovery/endurance   ☐ Aerobic/tempo   ☐ Anaerobic threshold

% time spent in target zone: _____

Injury or overtraining flags: Joint soreness   ☐ Yes   ☐ No

Moodiness   ☐ Yes   ☐ No

Slow recovery   ☐ Yes   ☐ No

Other: _____

Training and Nutrition Notes

Daily Training Log

Today's Goal   **Days until race:** _____

Today's Stats

Today's date:_____   Conditions:_____

Time of day: _____   Course: _____

Temperature:_____   Training partners: _____

80/20 Workout

☐ Intervals   ☐ Brick   ☐ Race simulation   ☐ Weakness   ☐ Power

Is this also a key workout?   ☐ Yes   ☐ No

Importance of 80/20 rule to goal: ☐ High   ☐ Moderate   ☐ Low

Workout Information

Discipline: ☐ Swim   ☐ Bike   ☐ Run   ☐ Other

Distances: _____   _____   _____   _____

Total time: _____   _____   _____   _____

Intensity: _____   _____   _____   _____

Other Details

Warm-up: _____   Cool-down: _____   Flexibility training: _____

Strength training: Weights _____   Sets _____   Reps _____

Results and Observations

Pace: _____   Splits: _____

Heart rate training: Resting heart rate: _____

Target zone: ☐ Recovery/endurance   ☐ Aerobic/tempo   ☐ Anaerobic threshold

% time spent in target zone: _____

Injury or overtraining flags: Joint soreness   ☐ Yes   ☐ No

                                                   Moodiness   ☐ Yes   ☐ No

                                                   Slow recovery   ☐ Yes   ☐ No

                                                   Other: _____

Training and Nutrition Notes

Daily Training Log

Today's Goal   **Days until race:** _____

Today's Stats

Today's date:_____   Conditions:_____

Time of day: _____   Course: _____

Temperature:_____   Training partners: _____

80/20 Workout

☐ Intervals   ☐ Brick   ☐ Race simulation   ☐ Weakness   ☐ Power

Is this also a key workout?   ☐ Yes   ☐ No

Importance of 80/20 rule to goal: ☐ High   ☐ Moderate   ☐ Low

Workout Information

Discipline: ☐ Swim   ☐ Bike   ☐ Run   ☐ Other

Distances: _____   _____   _____   _____

Total time: _____   _____   _____   _____

Intensity: _____   _____   _____   _____

Other Details

Warm-up: _____   Cool-down: _____   Flexibility training: _____

Strength training: Weights _____   Sets _____   Reps _____

Results and Observations

Pace: _____   Splits: _____

Heart rate training: Resting heart rate: _____

Target zone: ☐ Recovery/endurance   ☐ Aerobic/tempo   ☐ Anaerobic threshold

% time spent in target zone: _____

Injury or overtraining flags: Joint soreness   ☐ Yes   ☐ No

                                     Moodiness   ☐ Yes   ☐ No

                                     Slow recovery   ☐ Yes   ☐ No

                                     Other: _____

Training and Nutrition Notes

Weekly Planning Worksheet

This week's goal: _____

Training stage (circle one):   Base   STS   Peak   Tapering

	Workout activity	Distance or time	Type or intensity	Course	Notes
Monday					
Tuesday					
Wednesday					
Thursday					
Friday					
Saturday					
Sunday					

Target distance or time totals for this week:

Swim: _____   Bike: _____   Run: _____

Daily Training Log

Today's Goal

Days until race: _____

Today's Stats

Today's date:_____   Conditions:_____

Time of day: _____   Course: _____

Temperature:_____   Training partners: _____

80/20 Workout

☐ Intervals   ☐ Brick   ☐ Race simulation   ☐ Weakness   ☐ Power

Is this also a key workout?   ☐ Yes   ☐ No

Importance of 80/20 rule to goal: ☐ High   ☐ Moderate   ☐ Low

Workout Information

Discipline: ☐ Swim   ☐ Bike   ☐ Run   ☐ Other

Distances: _____   _____   _____   _____

Total time: _____   _____   _____   _____

Intensity: _____   _____   _____   _____

Other Details

Warm-up: _____   Cool-down: _____   Flexibility training: _____

Strength training: Weights _____   Sets _____   Reps _____

Results and Observations

Pace: _____   Splits: _____

Heart rate training: Resting heart rate: _____

Target zone: ☐ Recovery/endurance   ☐ Aerobic/tempo   ☐ Anaerobic threshold

% time spent in target zone: _____

Injury or overtraining flags: Joint soreness   ☐ Yes   ☐ No

                                                    Moodiness   ☐ Yes   ☐ No

                                                    Slow recovery   ☐ Yes   ☐ No

                                                    Other: _____

Training and Nutrition Notes

Daily Training Log

Today's Goal   *Days until race:* _____

Today's Stats

Today's date:_____   Conditions:_____

Time of day: _____   Course: _____

Temperature:_____   Training partners: _____

80/20 Workout

☐ Intervals   ☐ Brick   ☐ Race simulation   ☐ Weakness   ☐ Power

Is this also a key workout?   ☐ Yes   ☐ No

Importance of 80/20 rule to goal: ☐ High   ☐ Moderate   ☐ Low

Workout Information

Discipline:	☐ Swim	☐ Bike	☐ Run	☐ Other
Distances:	_____	_____	_____	_____
Total time:	_____	_____	_____	_____
Intensity:	_____	_____	_____	_____

Other Details

Warm-up: _____   Cool-down: _____   Flexibility training: _____

Strength training: Weights _____   Sets _____   Reps _____

Results and Observations

Pace: _____   Splits: _____

Heart rate training: Resting heart rate: _____

Target zone: ☐ Recovery/endurance   ☐ Aerobic/tempo   ☐ Anaerobic threshold

% time spent in target zone: _____

Injury or overtraining flags:	Joint soreness	☐ Yes	☐ No
	Moodiness	☐ Yes	☐ No
	Slow recovery	☐ Yes	☐ No
	Other: _____		

Training and Nutrition Notes

Daily Training Log

Today's Goal

Days until race: _____

Today's Stats

Today's date: _____   Conditions: _____

Time of day: _____   Course: _____

Temperature: _____   Training partners: _____

80/20 Workout

☐ Intervals   ☐ Brick   ☐ Race simulation   ☐ Weakness   ☐ Power

Is this also a key workout?   ☐ Yes   ☐ No

Importance of 80/20 rule to goal: ☐ High   ☐ Moderate   ☐ Low

Workout Information

Discipline: ☐ Swim   ☐ Bike   ☐ Run   ☐ Other

Distances: _____   _____   _____   _____

Total time: _____   _____   _____   _____

Intensity: _____   _____   _____   _____

Other Details

Warm-up: _____   Cool-down: _____   Flexibility training: _____

Strength training: Weights _____   Sets _____   Reps _____

Results and Observations

Pace: _____   Splits: _____

Heart rate training: Resting heart rate: _____

Target zone: ☐ Recovery/endurance   ☐ Aerobic/tempo   ☐ Anaerobic threshold

% time spent in target zone: _____

Injury or overtraining flags: Joint soreness   ☐ Yes   ☐ No

                                       Moodiness   ☐ Yes   ☐ No

                                       Slow recovery   ☐ Yes   ☐ No

                                       Other: _____

Training and Nutrition Notes

Daily Training Log

Today's Goal   *Days until race:* _____

Today's Stats

Today's date: _____   Conditions: _____

Time of day: _____   Course: _____

Temperature: _____   Training partners: _____

80/20 Workout

☐ Intervals   ☐ Brick   ☐ Race simulation   ☐ Weakness   ☐ Power

Is this also a key workout?   ☐ Yes   ☐ No

Importance of 80/20 rule to goal: ☐ High   ☐ Moderate   ☐ Low

Workout Information

Discipline: ☐ Swim   ☐ Bike   ☐ Run   ☐ Other

Distances: _____   _____   _____   _____

Total time: _____   _____   _____   _____

Intensity: _____   _____   _____   _____

Other Details

Warm-up: _____   Cool-down: _____   Flexibility training: _____

Strength training: Weights _____   Sets _____   Reps _____

Results and Observations

Pace: _____   Splits: _____

Heart rate training: Resting heart rate: _____

Target zone: ☐ Recovery/endurance   ☐ Aerobic/tempo   ☐ Anaerobic threshold

% time spent in target zone: _____

Injury or overtraining flags: Joint soreness   ☐ Yes   ☐ No

Moodiness   ☐ Yes   ☐ No

Slow recovery   ☐ Yes   ☐ No

Other: _____

Training and Nutrition Notes

Daily Training Log

Today's Goal

Today's Stats

Today's date: _____   Conditions: _____

Time of day: _____   Course: _____

Temperature: _____   Training partners: _____

80/20 Workout

☐ Intervals   ☐ Brick   ☐ Race simulation   ☐ Weakness   ☐ Power

Is this also a key workout?   ☐ Yes   ☐ No

Importance of 80/20 rule to goal: ☐ High   ☐ Moderate   ☐ Low

Workout Information

Discipline: ☐ Swim   ☐ Bike   ☐ Run   ☐ Other

Distances: _____   _____   _____   _____

Total time: _____   _____   _____   _____

Intensity: _____   _____   _____   _____

Other Details

Warm-up: _____   Cool-down: _____   Flexibility training: _____

Strength training: Weights _____   Sets _____   Reps _____

Results and Observations

Pace: _____   Splits: _____

Heart rate training: Resting heart rate: _____

Target zone: ☐ Recovery/endurance   ☐ Aerobic/tempo   ☐ Anaerobic threshold

% time spent in target zone: _____

Injury or overtraining flags: Joint soreness   ☐ Yes   ☐ No

Moodiness   ☐ Yes   ☐ No

Slow recovery   ☐ Yes   ☐ No

Other: _____

Training and Nutrition Notes

Daily Training Log

Today's Goal   ***Days until race:*** _____

Today's Stats

Today's date:_____   Conditions:_____

Time of day: _____   Course: _____

Temperature:_____   Training partners: _____

80/20 Workout

☐ Intervals   ☐ Brick   ☐ Race simulation   ☐ Weakness   ☐ Power

Is this also a key workout?   ☐ Yes   ☐ No

Importance of 80/20 rule to goal: ☐ High   ☐ Moderate   ☐ Low

Workout Information

Discipline: ☐ Swim   ☐ Bike   ☐ Run   ☐ Other

Distances: _____   _____   _____   _____

Total time: _____   _____   _____   _____

Intensity: _____   _____   _____   _____

Other Details

Warm-up: _____   Cool-down: _____   Flexibility training: _____

Strength training: Weights _____   Sets _____   Reps _____

Results and Observations

Pace: _____   Splits: _____

Heart rate training: Resting heart rate: _____

Target zone: ☐ Recovery/endurance   ☐ Aerobic/tempo   ☐ Anaerobic threshold

% time spent in target zone: _____

Injury or overtraining flags: Joint soreness   ☐ Yes   ☐ No

                                             Moodiness   ☐ Yes   ☐ No

                                             Slow recovery   ☐ Yes   ☐ No

                                             Other: _____

Training and Nutrition Notes

Daily Training Log

Today's Goal

Days until race: _____

Today's Stats

Today's date: _____   Conditions: _____

Time of day: _____   Course: _____

Temperature: _____   Training partners: _____

80/20 Workout

☐ Intervals   ☐ Brick   ☐ Race simulation   ☐ Weakness   ☐ Power

Is this also a key workout?   ☐ Yes   ☐ No

Importance of 80/20 rule to goal: ☐ High   ☐ Moderate   ☐ Low

Workout Information

Discipline:	☐ Swim	☐ Bike	☐ Run	☐ Other
Distances:	_____	_____	_____	_____
Total time:	_____	_____	_____	_____
Intensity:	_____	_____	_____	_____

Other Details

Warm-up: _____   Cool-down: _____   Flexibility training: _____

Strength training: Weights _____   Sets _____   Reps _____

Results and Observations

Pace: _____   Splits: _____

Heart rate training: Resting heart rate: _____

Target zone: ☐ Recovery/endurance   ☐ Aerobic/tempo   ☐ Anaerobic threshold

% time spent in target zone: _____

Injury or overtraining flags: Joint soreness   ☐ Yes   ☐ No

Moodiness   ☐ Yes   ☐ No

Slow recovery   ☐ Yes   ☐ No

Other: _____

Training and Nutrition Notes

Weekly Planning Worksheet

This week's goal: _____

Training stage (circle one):   Base   STS   Peak   Tapering

	Workout activity	Distance or time	Type or intensity	Course	Notes
Monday					
Tuesday					
Wednesday					
Thursday					
Friday					
Saturday					
Sunday					

Target distance or time totals for this week:

Swim: _____   Bike: _____   Run: _____

Daily Training Log

Today's Goal
Days until race: _____

Today's Stats
Today's date: _____   Conditions: _____

Time of day: _____   Course: _____

Temperature: _____   Training partners: _____

80/20 Workout
☐ Intervals   ☐ Brick   ☐ Race simulation   ☐ Weakness   ☐ Power

Is this also a key workout?   ☐ Yes   ☐ No

Importance of 80/20 rule to goal: ☐ High   ☐ Moderate   ☐ Low

Workout Information
Discipline: ☐ Swim   ☐ Bike   ☐ Run   ☐ Other

Distances: _____   _____   _____   _____

Total time: _____   _____   _____   _____

Intensity: _____   _____   _____   _____

Other Details
Warm-up: _____   Cool-down: _____   Flexibility training: _____

Strength training: Weights _____   Sets _____   Reps _____

Results and Observations
Pace: _____   Splits: _____

Heart rate training: Resting heart rate: _____

Target zone: ☐ Recovery/endurance   ☐ Aerobic/tempo   ☐ Anaerobic threshold

% time spent in target zone: _____

Injury or overtraining flags: Joint soreness   ☐ Yes   ☐ No

     Moodiness   ☐ Yes   ☐ No

     Slow recovery   ☐ Yes   ☐ No

     Other: _____

Training and Nutrition Notes

Daily Training Log

Today's Goal   *Days until race:* _____

Today's Stats

Today's date:_____   Conditions:_____

Time of day: _____   Course: _____

Temperature:_____   Training partners: _____

80/20 Workout

☐ Intervals   ☐ Brick   ☐ Race simulation   ☐ Weakness   ☐ Power

Is this also a key workout?   ☐ Yes   ☐ No

Importance of 80/20 rule to goal: ☐ High   ☐ Moderate   ☐ Low

Workout Information

Discipline: ☐ Swim   ☐ Bike   ☐ Run   ☐ Other

Distances: _____   _____   _____   _____

Total time: _____   _____   _____   _____

Intensity: _____   _____   _____   _____

Other Details

Warm-up: _____   Cool-down: _____   Flexibility training: _____

Strength training: Weights _____   Sets _____   Reps _____

Results and Observations

Pace: _____   Splits: _____

Heart rate training: Resting heart rate: _____

Target zone: ☐ Recovery/endurance   ☐ Aerobic/tempo   ☐ Anaerobic threshold

% time spent in target zone: _____

Injury or overtraining flags: Joint soreness   ☐ Yes   ☐ No

Moodiness   ☐ Yes   ☐ No

Slow recovery   ☐ Yes   ☐ No

Other: _____

Training and Nutrition Notes

Daily Training Log

Today's Goal

Days until race: _____

Today's Stats

Today's date: _____   Conditions: _____

Time of day: _____   Course: _____

Temperature: _____   Training partners: _____

80/20 Workout

☐ Intervals   ☐ Brick   ☐ Race simulation   ☐ Weakness   ☐ Power

Is this also a key workout?   ☐ Yes   ☐ No

Importance of 80/20 rule to goal: ☐ High   ☐ Moderate   ☐ Low

Workout Information

Discipline:	☐ Swim	☐ Bike	☐ Run	☐ Other
Distances:	_____	_____	_____	_____
Total time:	_____	_____	_____	_____
Intensity:	_____	_____	_____	_____

Other Details

Warm-up: _____   Cool-down: _____   Flexibility training: _____

Strength training: Weights _____   Sets _____   Reps _____

Results and Observations

Pace: _____   Splits: _____

Heart rate training: Resting heart rate: _____

Target zone: ☐ Recovery/endurance   ☐ Aerobic/tempo   ☐ Anaerobic threshold

% time spent in target zone: _____

Injury or overtraining flags:	Joint soreness	☐ Yes	☐ No
	Moodiness	☐ Yes	☐ No
	Slow recovery	☐ Yes	☐ No
	Other: _____		

Training and Nutrition Notes

Daily Training Log

Today's Goal   *Days until race:* _____

Today's Stats

Today's date: _____   Conditions: _____

Time of day: _____   Course: _____

Temperature: _____   Training partners: _____

80/20 Workout

☐ Intervals   ☐ Brick   ☐ Race simulation   ☐ Weakness   ☐ Power

Is this also a key workout?   ☐ Yes   ☐ No

Importance of 80/20 rule to goal: ☐ High   ☐ Moderate   ☐ Low

Workout Information

Discipline: ☐ Swim   ☐ Bike   ☐ Run   ☐ Other

Distances: _____   _____   _____   _____

Total time: _____   _____   _____   _____

Intensity: _____   _____   _____   _____

Other Details

Warm-up: _____   Cool-down: _____   Flexibility training: _____

Strength training: Weights _____   Sets _____   Reps _____

Results and Observations

Pace: _____   Splits: _____

Heart rate training: Resting heart rate: _____

Target zone: ☐ Recovery/endurance   ☐ Aerobic/tempo   ☐ Anaerobic threshold

% time spent in target zone: _____

Injury or overtraining flags: Joint soreness   ☐ Yes   ☐ No

                                      Moodiness   ☐ Yes   ☐ No

                                      Slow recovery   ☐ Yes   ☐ No

                                      Other: _____

Training and Nutrition Notes

Daily Training Log

Today's Goal

Days until race: _____

Today's Stats

Today's date: _____   Conditions: _____

Time of day: _____   Course _____

Temperature: _____   Training partners: _____

80/20 Workout

☐ Intervals   ☐ Brick   ☐ Race simulation   ☐ Weakness   ☐ Power

Is this also a key workout?   ☐ Yes   ☐ No

Importance of 80/20 rule to goal: ☐ High   ☐ Moderate   ☐ Low

Workout Information

Discipline: ☐ Swim   ☐ Bike   ☐ Run   ☐ Other

Distances: _____   _____   _____   _____

Total time: _____   _____   _____   _____

Intensity: _____   _____   _____   _____

Other Details

Warm-up: _____   Cool-down: _____   Flexibility training: _____

Strength training: Weights _____   Sets _____   Reps _____

Results and Observations

Pace: _____   Splits: _____

Heart rate training: Resting heart rate: _____

Target zone: ☐ Recovery/endurance   ☐ Aerobic/tempo   ☐ Anaerobic threshold

% time spent in target zone: _____

Injury or overtraining flags: Joint soreness   ☐ Yes   ☐ No

                                                    Moodiness   ☐ Yes   ☐ No

                                                    Slow recovery   ☐ Yes   ☐ No

                                                    Other: _____

Training and Nutrition Notes

Daily Training Log

Today's Goal   **Days until race:** _____

Today's Stats

Today's date:_____   Conditions:_____

Time of day: _____   Course: _____

Temperature:_____   Training partners: _____

80/20 Workout

☐ Intervals   ☐ Brick   ☐ Race simulation   ☐ Weakness   ☐ Power

Is this also a key workout?   ☐ Yes   ☐ No

Importance of 80/20 rule to goal: ☐ High   ☐ Moderate   ☐ Low

Workout Information

Discipline:	☐ Swim	☐ Bike	☐ Run	☐ Other
Distances:	_____	_____	_____	_____
Total time:	_____	_____	_____	_____
Intensity:	_____	_____	_____	_____

Other Details

Warm-up: _____   Cool-down: _____   Flexibility training: _____

Strength training: Weights _____   Sets _____   Reps _____

Results and Observations

Pace: _____   Splits: _____

Heart rate training: Resting heart rate: _____

Target zone: ☐ Recovery/endurance   ☐ Aerobic/tempo   ☐ Anaerobic threshold

% time spent in target zone: _____

Injury or overtraining flags: Joint soreness   ☐ Yes   ☐ No

                                      Moodiness   ☐ Yes   ☐ No

                                      Slow recovery   ☐ Yes   ☐ No

                                      Other: _____

Training and Nutrition Notes

Daily Training Log

Today's Goal

Days until race: _____

Today's Stats

Today's date: _____   Conditions: _____

Time of day: _____   Course: _____

Temperature: _____   Training partners: _____

80/20 Workout

☐ Intervals   ☐ Brick   ☐ Race simulation   ☐ Weakness   ☐ Power

Is this also a key workout?   ☐ Yes   ☐ No

Importance of 80/20 rule to goal: ☐ High   ☐ Moderate   ☐ Low

Workout Information

Discipline:	☐ Swim	☐ Bike	☐ Run	☐ Other
Distances:	_____	_____	_____	_____
Total time:	_____	_____	_____	_____
Intensity:	_____	_____	_____	_____

Other Details

Warm-up: _____   Cool-down: _____   Flexibility training: _____

Strength training: Weights _____   Sets _____   Reps _____

Results and Observations

Pace: _____   Splits: _____

Heart rate training: Resting heart rate: _____

Target zone: ☐ Recovery/endurance   ☐ Aerobic/tempo   ☐ Anaerobic threshold

% time spent in target zone: _____

Injury or overtraining flags:

	Joint soreness	☐ Yes	☐ No
	Moodiness	☐ Yes	☐ No
	Slow recovery	☐ Yes	☐ No
	Other: _____		

Training and Nutrition Notes

Weekly Planning Worksheet

This week's goal: _____

Training stage (circle one):   Base   STS   Peak   Tapering

	Workout activity	Distance or time	Type or intensity	Course	Notes
Monday					
Tuesday					
Wednesday					
Thursday					
Friday					
Saturday					
Sunday					

Target distance or time totals for this week:

Swim: _____   Bike: _____   Run: _____

Daily Training Log

Today's Goal   **Days until race:** _____

Today's Stats

Today's date:_____   Conditions:_____

Time of day: _____   Course: _____

Temperature:_____   Training partners: _____

80/20 Workout

☐ Intervals   ☐ Brick   ☐ Race simulation   ☐ Weakness   ☐ Power

Is this also a key workout?   ☐ Yes   ☐ No

Importance of 80/20 rule to goal: ☐ High   ☐ Moderate   ☐ Low

Workout Information

Discipline: ☐ Swim   ☐ Bike   ☐ Run   ☐ Other

Distances: _____   _____   _____   _____

Total time: _____   _____   _____   _____

Intensity: _____   _____   _____   _____

Other Details

Warm-up: _____   Cool-down: _____   Flexibility training: _____

Strength training: Weights _____   Sets _____   Reps _____

Results and Observations

Pace: _____   Splits: _____

Heart rate training: Resting heart rate: _____

Target zone: ☐ Recovery/endurance   ☐ Aerobic/tempo   ☐ Anaerobic threshold

% time spent in target zone: _____

Injury or overtraining flags: Joint soreness   ☐ Yes   ☐ No

                                      Moodiness   ☐ Yes   ☐ No

                                      Slow recovery   ☐ Yes   ☐ No

                                      Other: _____

Training and Nutrition Notes

Daily Training Log

Today's Goal   *Days until race:* _____

Today's Stats

Today's date:_____   Conditions:_____

Time of day: _____   Course: _____

Temperature:_____   Training partners: _____

80/20 Workout

☐ Intervals   ☐ Brick   ☐ Race simulation   ☐ Weakness   ☐ Power

Is this also a key workout?   ☐ Yes   ☐ No

Importance of 80/20 rule to goal: ☐ High   ☐ Moderate   ☐ Low

Workout Information

Discipline: ☐ Swim   ☐ Bike   ☐ Run   ☐ Other

Distances: _____   _____   _____   _____

Total time: _____   _____   _____   _____

Intensity: _____   _____   _____   _____

Other Details

Warm-up: _____   Cool-down: _____   Flexibility training: _____

Strength training: Weights _____   Sets _____   Reps _____

Results and Observations

Pace: _____   Splits: _____

Heart rate training: Resting heart rate: _____

Target zone: ☐ Recovery/endurance   ☐ Aerobic/tempo   ☐ Anaerobic threshold

% time spent in target zone: _____

Injury or overtraining flags: Joint soreness   ☐ Yes   ☐ No

Moodiness   ☐ Yes   ☐ No

Slow recovery   ☐ Yes   ☐ No

Other: _____

Training and Nutrition Notes

Daily Training Log

Today's Goal   *Days until race:* _____

Today's Stats

Today's date:_____   Conditions:_____

Time of day: _____   Course: _____

Temperature:_____   Training partners: _____

80/20 Workout

☐ Intervals   ☐ Brick   ☐ Race simulation   ☐ Weakness   ☐ Power

Is this also a key workout?   ☐ Yes   ☐ No

Importance of 80/20 rule to goal: ☐ High   ☐ Moderate   ☐ Low

Workout Information

Discipline: ☐ Swim   ☐ Bike   ☐ Run   ☐ Other

Distances: _____   _____   _____   _____

Total time: _____   _____   _____   _____

Intensity: _____   _____   _____   _____

Other Details

Warm-up: _____   Cool-down: _____   Flexibility training: _____

Strength training: Weights _____   Sets _____   Reps _____

Results and Observations

Pace: _____   Splits: _____

Heart rate training: Resting heart rate: _____

Target zone: ☐ Recovery/endurance   ☐ Aerobic/tempo   ☐ Anaerobic threshold

% time spent in target zone: _____

Injury or overtraining flags: Joint soreness   ☐ Yes   ☐ No

                                       Moodiness   ☐ Yes   ☐ No

                                       Slow recovery   ☐ Yes   ☐ No

                                       Other: _____

Training and Nutrition Notes

Daily Training Log

Today's Goal

Days until race: _____

Today's Stats

Today's date:_____   Conditions:_____

Time of day: _____   Course: _____

Temperature:_____   Training partners: _____

80/20 Workout

☐ Intervals   ☐ Brick   ☐ Race simulation   ☐ Weakness   ☐ Power

Is this also a key workout?   ☐ Yes   ☐ No

Importance of 80/20 rule to goal: ☐ High   ☐ Moderate   ☐ Low

Workout Information

Discipline:	☐ Swim	☐ Bike	☐ Run	☐ Other
Distances:	_____	_____	_____	_____
Total time:	_____	_____	_____	_____
Intensity:	_____	_____	_____	_____

Other Details

Warm-up: _____   Cool-down: _____   Flexibility training: _____

Strength training: Weights _____   Sets _____   Reps _____

Results and Observations

Pace: _____   Splits: _____

Heart rate training: Resting heart rate: _____

Target zone: ☐ Recovery/endurance   ☐ Aerobic/tempo   ☐ Anaerobic threshold

% time spent in target zone: _____

Injury or overtraining flags: Joint soreness   ☐ Yes   ☐ No

Moodiness   ☐ Yes   ☐ No

Slow recovery   ☐ Yes   ☐ No

Other: _____

Training and Nutrition Notes

Daily Training Log

Today's Goal

Days until race: _____

Today's Stats

Today's date: _____   Conditions: _____

Time of day: _____   Course: _____

Temperature: _____   Training partners: _____

80/20 Workout

☐ Intervals   ☐ Brick   ☐ Race simulation   ☐ Weakness   ☐ Power

Is this also a key workout?   ☐ Yes   ☐ No

Importance of 80/20 rule to goal: ☐ High   ☐ Moderate   ☐ Low

Workout Information

Discipline:	☐ Swim	☐ Bike	☐ Run	☐ Other
Distances:	_____	_____	_____	_____
Total time:	_____	_____	_____	_____
Intensity:	_____	_____	_____	_____

Other Details

Warm-up: _____   Cool-down: _____   Flexibility training: _____

Strength training: Weights _____   Sets _____   Reps _____

Results and Observations

Pace: _____   Splits: _____

Heart rate training: Resting heart rate: _____

Target zone: ☐ Recovery/endurance   ☐ Aerobic/tempo   ☐ Anaerobic threshold

% time spent in target zone: _____

Injury or overtraining flags:	Joint soreness	☐ Yes	☐ No
	Moodiness	☐ Yes	☐ No
	Slow recovery	☐ Yes	☐ No
	Other: _____		

Training and Nutrition Notes

Daily Training Log

Today's Goal   ***Days until race:*** _____

Today's Stats

Today's date:_____   Conditions:_____

Time of day: _____   Course: _____

Temperature:_____   Training partners: _____

80/20 Workout

☐ Intervals   ☐ Brick   ☐ Race simulation   ☐ Weakness   ☐ Power

Is this also a key workout?   ☐ Yes   ☐ No

Importance of 80/20 rule to goal: ☐ High   ☐ Moderate   ☐ Low

Workout Information

Discipline: ☐ Swim   ☐ Bike   ☐ Run   ☐ Other

Distances: _____   _____   _____   _____

Total time: _____   _____   _____   _____

Intensity: _____   _____   _____   _____

Other Details

Warm-up: _____   Cool-down: _____   Flexibility training: _____

Strength training: Weights _____   Sets _____   Reps _____

Results and Observations

Pace: _____   Splits: _____

Heart rate training: Resting heart rate: _____

Target zone: ☐ Recovery/endurance   ☐ Aerobic/tempo   ☐ Anaerobic threshold

% time spent in target zone: _____

Injury or overtraining flags: Joint soreness   ☐ Yes   ☐ No

                                         Moodiness   ☐ Yes   ☐ No

                                         Slow recovery   ☐ Yes   ☐ No

                                         Other: _____

Training and Nutrition Notes

Daily Training Log

Today's Goal

Days until race: _____

Today's Stats

Today's date: _____   Conditions: _____

Time of day: _____   Course: _____

Temperature: _____   Training partners: _____

80/20 Workout

☐ Intervals   ☐ Brick   ☐ Race simulation   ☐ Weakness   ☐ Power

Is this also a key workout?   ☐ Yes   ☐ No

Importance of 80/20 rule to goal: ☐ High   ☐ Moderate   ☐ Low

Workout Information

Discipline:	☐ Swim	☐ Bike	☐ Run	☐ Other
Distances:	_____	_____	_____	_____
Total time:	_____	_____	_____	_____
Intensity:	_____	_____	_____	_____

Other Details

Warm-up: _____   Cool-down: _____   Flexibility training: _____

Strength training: Weights _____   Sets _____   Reps _____

Results and Observations

Pace: _____   Splits: _____

Heart rate training: Resting heart rate: _____

Target zone: ☐ Recovery/endurance   ☐ Aerobic/tempo   ☐ Anaerobic threshold

% time spent in target zone: _____

Injury or overtraining flags: Joint soreness   ☐ Yes   ☐ No

Moodiness   ☐ Yes   ☐ No

Slow recovery   ☐ Yes   ☐ No

Other: _____

Training and Nutrition Notes

Weekly Planning Worksheet

This week's goal: _____

Training stage (circle one): Base STS Peak Tapering

	Workout activity	Distance or time	Type or intensity	Course	Notes
Monday					
Tuesday					
Wednesday					
Thursday					
Friday					
Saturday					
Sunday					

Target distance or time totals for this week:

Swim: _____   Bike: _____   Run: _____

Daily Training Log

Today's Goal

Days until race: _____

Today's Stats

Today's date: _____

Time of day: _____

Temperature: _____

Conditions: _____

Course: _____

Training partners: _____

80/20 Workout

☐ Intervals   ☐ Brick   ☐ Race simulation   ☐ Weakness   ☐ Power

Is this also a key workout?   ☐ Yes   ☐ No

Importance of 80/20 rule to goal: ☐ High   ☐ Moderate   ☐ Low

Workout Information

Discipline: ☐ Swim   ☐ Bike   ☐ Run   ☐ Other

Distances: _____   _____   _____   _____

Total time: _____   _____   _____   _____

Intensity: _____   _____   _____   _____

Other Details

Warm-up: _____   Cool-down: _____   Flexibility training: _____

Strength training: Weights _____   Sets _____   Reps _____

Results and Observations

Pace: _____   Splits: _____

Heart rate training: Resting heart rate: _____

Target zone: ☐ Recovery/endurance   ☐ Aerobic/tempo   ☐ Anaerobic threshold

% time spent in target zone: _____

Injury or overtraining flags: Joint soreness   ☐ Yes   ☐ No

Moodiness   ☐ Yes   ☐ No

Slow recovery   ☐ Yes   ☐ No

Other: _____

Training and Nutrition Notes

Daily Training Log

Today's Goal

Days until race: _____

Today's Stats

Today's date:_____   Conditions:_____

Time of day: _____   Course: _____

Temperature:_____   Training partners: _____

80/20 Workout

☐ Intervals   ☐ Brick   ☐ Race simulation   ☐ Weakness   ☐ Power

Is this also a key workout?   ☐ Yes   ☐ No

Importance of 80/20 rule to goal: ☐ High   ☐ Moderate   ☐ Low

Workout Information

Discipline:	☐ Swim	☐ Bike	☐ Run	☐ Other
Distances:	_____	_____	_____	_____
Total time:	_____	_____	_____	_____
Intensity:	_____	_____	_____	_____

Other Details

Warm-up: _____   Cool-down: _____   Flexibility training: _____

Strength training: Weights _____   Sets _____   Reps _____

Results and Observations

Pace: _____   Splits: _____

Heart rate training: Resting heart rate: _____

Target zone: ☐ Recovery/endurance   ☐ Aerobic/tempo   ☐ Anaerobic threshold

% time spent in target zone: _____

Injury or overtraining flags: Joint soreness   ☐ Yes   ☐ No

Moodiness   ☐ Yes   ☐ No

Slow recovery   ☐ Yes   ☐ No

Other: _____

Training and Nutrition Notes

Daily Training Log

Today's Goal   ***Days until race:*** _____

Today's Stats

Today's date: _____   Conditions: _____

Time of day: _____   Course: _____

Temperature: _____   Training partners: _____

80/20 Workout

☐ Intervals   ☐ Brick   ☐ Race simulation   ☐ Weakness   ☐ Power

Is this also a key workout?   ☐ Yes   ☐ No

Importance of 80/20 rule to goal: ☐ High   ☐ Moderate   ☐ Low

Workout Information

Discipline:	☐ Swim	☐ Bike	☐ Run	☐ Other
Distances:	_____	_____	_____	_____
Total time:	_____	_____	_____	_____
Intensity:	_____	_____	_____	_____

Other Details

Warm-up: _____   Cool-down: _____   Flexibility training: _____

Strength training: Weights _____   Sets _____   Reps _____

Results and Observations

Pace: _____   Splits: _____

Heart rate training: Resting heart rate: _____

Target zone: ☐ Recovery/endurance   ☐ Aerobic/tempo   ☐ Anaerobic threshold

% time spent in target zone: _____

Injury or overtraining flags: Joint soreness   ☐ Yes   ☐ No

                                         Moodiness   ☐ Yes   ☐ No

                                         Slow recovery   ☐ Yes   ☐ No

                                         Other: _____

Training and Nutrition Notes

Daily Training Log

Today's Goal   ***Days until race:*** _____

Today's Stats

Today's date:_____   Conditions:_____

Time of day: _____   Course: _____

Temperature:_____   Training partners: _____

80/20 Workout

☐ Intervals   ☐ Brick   ☐ Race simulation   ☐ Weakness   ☐ Power

Is this also a key workout?   ☐ Yes   ☐ No

Importance of 80/20 rule to goal: ☐ High   ☐ Moderate   ☐ Low

Workout Information

Discipline:	☐ Swim	☐ Bike	☐ Run	☐ Other
Distances:	_____	_____	_____	_____
Total time:	_____	_____	_____	_____
Intensity:	_____	_____	_____	_____

Other Details

Warm-up: _____   Cool-down: _____   Flexibility training: _____

Strength training: Weights _____   Sets _____   Reps _____

Results and Observations

Pace: _____   Splits: _____

Heart rate training: Resting heart rate: _____

Target zone: ☐ Recovery/endurance   ☐ Aerobic/tempo   ☐ Anaerobic threshold

% time spent in target zone: _____

Injury or overtraining flags: Joint soreness   ☐ Yes   ☐ No

                                            Moodiness   ☐ Yes   ☐ No

                                            Slow recovery   ☐ Yes   ☐ No

                                            Other: _____

Training and Nutrition Notes

Daily Training Log

Today's Goal   *Days until race:* _____

Today's Stats

Today's date: _____   Conditions: _____

Time of day: _____   Course: _____

Temperature: _____   Training partners: _____

80/20 Workout

☐ Intervals   ☐ Brick   ☐ Race simulation   ☐ Weakness   ☐ Power

Is this also a key workout?   ☐ Yes   ☐ No

Importance of 80/20 rule to goal: ☐ High   ☐ Moderate   ☐ Low

Workout Information

Discipline: ☐ Swim   ☐ Bike   ☐ Run   ☐ Other

Distances: _____   _____   _____   _____

Total time: _____   _____   _____   _____

Intensity: _____   _____   _____   _____

Other Details

Warm-up: _____   Cool-down: _____   Flexibility training: _____

Strength training: Weights _____   Sets _____   Reps _____

Results and Observations

Pace: _____   Splits: _____

Heart rate training: Resting heart rate: _____

Target zone: ☐ Recovery/endurance   ☐ Aerobic/tempo   ☐ Anaerobic threshold

% time spent in target zone: _____

Injury or overtraining flags: Joint soreness   ☐ Yes   ☐ No

                                          Moodiness   ☐ Yes   ☐ No

                                          Slow recovery   ☐ Yes   ☐ No

                                          Other: _____

Training and Nutrition Notes

Daily Training Log

Today's Goal   *Days until race:* _____

Today's Stats

Today's date:_____   Conditions:_____

Time of day: _____   Course: _____

Temperature:_____   Training partners: _____

80/20 Workout

☐ Intervals   ☐ Brick   ☐ Race simulation   ☐ Weakness   ☐ Power

Is this also a key workout?   ☐ Yes   ☐ No

Importance of 80/20 rule to goal: ☐ High   ☐ Moderate   ☐ Low

Workout Information

Discipline: ☐ Swim   ☐ Bike   ☐ Run   ☐ Other

Distances: _____   _____   _____   _____

Total time: _____   _____   _____   _____

Intensity: _____   _____   _____   _____

Other Details

Warm-up: _____   Cool-down: _____   Flexibility training: _____

Strength training: Weights _____   Sets _____   Reps _____

Results and Observations

Pace: _____   Splits: _____

Heart rate training: Resting heart rate: _____

Target zone: ☐ Recovery/endurance   ☐ Aerobic/tempo   ☐ Anaerobic threshold

% time spent in target zone: _____

Injury or overtraining flags: Joint soreness   ☐ Yes   ☐ No

                                      Moodiness   ☐ Yes   ☐ No

                                      Slow recovery   ☐ Yes   ☐ No

                                      Other: _____

Training and Nutrition Notes

Daily Training Log

Today's Goal

Days until race: _____

Today's Stats

Today's date: _____   Conditions: _____

Time of day: _____   Course: _____

Temperature: _____   Training partners: _____

80/20 Workout

☐ Intervals   ☐ Brick   ☐ Race simulation   ☐ Weakness   ☐ Power

Is this also a key workout?   ☐ Yes   ☐ No

Importance of 80/20 rule to goal: ☐ High   ☐ Moderate   ☐ Low

Workout Information

Discipline: ☐ Swim   ☐ Bike   ☐ Run   ☐ Other

Distances: _____   _____   _____   _____

Total time: _____   _____   _____   _____

Intensity: _____   _____   _____   _____

Other Details

Warm-up: _____   Cool-down: _____   Flexibility training: _____

Strength training: Weights _____   Sets _____   Reps _____

Results and Observations

Pace: _____   Splits: _____

Heart rate training: Resting heart rate: _____

Target zone: ☐ Recovery/endurance   ☐ Aerobic/tempo   ☐ Anaerobic threshold

% time spent in target zone: _____

Injury or overtraining flags: Joint soreness   ☐ Yes   ☐ No

     Moodiness   ☐ Yes   ☐ No

     Slow recovery   ☐ Yes   ☐ No

     Other: _____

Training and Nutrition Notes

Monthly Training Summary (Weeks 1-4)

Month: _____	Swim Totals	Bike Totals	Run Totals
Week 1			
Week 2			
Week 3			
Week 4			
This month's totals			
Last month's totals			
YTD (or season) totals			

Monthly Training Summary (Weeks 5-8)

Month: _____	Swim Totals	Bike Totals	Run Totals
Week 5			
Week 6			
Week 7			
Week 8			
This month's totals			
Last month's totals			
YTD (or season) totals			

Notes

Notes

Notes

Notes

References

Cooper, K.H. 1968. A means of assessing maximal oxygen uptake. *Journal of the American Medical Association* 203:201-204.

Endurance Research Board. 2004. Recovery recipe for success. [Online]. www.trifuel.com/triathlon/nutrition/recovery-recipe-for-success-000398.php. Accessed November 10, 2005.

Galloway, Jeff. 1984. *Galloway's Book on Running*. Bolinas, CA: Shelter.

Kifer, Ken. 2002. Auto costs versus bike costs. [Online]. www.kenkifer.com/bikepages/advocacy/autocost.htm. Accessed November 10, 2005.

Newby-Fraser, Paula. 1995. *Peak Fitness for Women*. Champaign, IL: Human Kinetics.

Neary J.P., T.P. Martin, D.C. Reid, R. Burnham, and H.A. Quinney. 1992. The effects of reduced exercise duration taper programme on performance and muscle enzymes of endurance cyclists. *European Journal of Applied Physiology* 65:30-36.

Sheehan, George. 1989. *Personal Best*. Emmaus, PA: Rodale Press.

Vleck, V.E., and G. Garbutt. 1998. Injury and training characteristics of male elite, development squad, and club triathletes. *International Journal of Sports Medicine* 19:8-42.

Index

Note: The italicized *t* following page numbers refers to tables.

About the Author

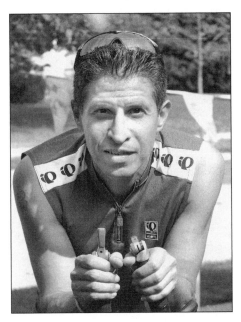

John M. Mora is a prolific sports, health and fitness, and medical writer. He is a former contributing editor to *Triathlete* and currently serves as the running columnist and triathlon feature writer for *Windy City Sports*. He has written more than 400 articles for national magazines, including *American Health, Women's Sports & Fitness,* and *Runner's World*. He also coauthored *Paula Newby-Fraser's Peak Fitness for Women* (Human Kinetics, 1995) with eight-time Gatorade Hawaii Ironman Triathlon world champion Paula Newby-Fraser. Mora's second book with Human Kinetics, *Triathlon 101*, has sold more than 60,000 copies worldwide and has been translated into two foreign languages. Born in Chicago, Mora has competed around the country in 10 marathons, 70 running and cycling events, and 80 triathlons of various distances, from sprint to Ironman. He currently owns Creative3, a marketing business specializing in the health, fitness, and medical industries. Mora lives and trains in Plainfield, Illinois, a suburb of Chicago.

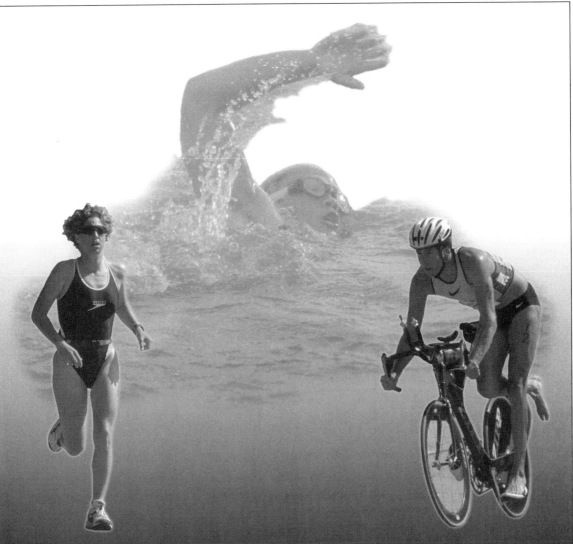